History of the Body

Theory and History
Series Editor: Donald MacRaild

Published

History of the Body

Willemijn Ruberg

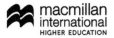 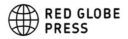

First published 2020 by
RED GLOBE PRESS

Red Globe Press in the UK is an imprint of Springer Nature Limited, registered in England, company number 785998, of 4 Crinan Street, London N1 9XW.

Red Globe Press® is a registered trademark in the United States, the United Kingdom, Europe and other countries.

ISBN 978-1-352-00771-8 hardback
ISBN 978-1-352-00768-8 paperback

This book is printed on paper suitable for recycling and made from fully managed and sustained forest sources. Logging, pulping and manufacturing processes are expected to conform to the environmental regulations of the country of origin.

A catalogue record for this book is available from the British Library.

A catalog record for this book is available from the Library of Congress.

Contents

Introduction

▶ The rise of the history of the body

The history of the body as a separate field was shaped in the 1980s and 1990s. This new attention to the body has been variously referred to as the corporeal, bodily, or **somatic turn**. Before this corporeal turn, historians had, as the French medievalist Jacques le Goff put it, written the histories of men (and to a lesser extent, women) 'without bodies', that is histories of disembodied people's thoughts and ideas.[1] The body in history had mostly been discussed by historians of medicine, who, however, assumed the body to be an unchanging biological entity. It was the British historian Roy Porter who first provided an overview of the new history of the body in 1991, in a volume edited by Peter Burke that distanced itself from a more traditional history focused on the 'objective' reconstruction of political events. The new history, by contrast, was concerned with socio-economic, cultural, and political dimensions, an analysis of structures and daily life 'from below', all of this based on an interdisciplinary analysis of a variety of primary sources and keen to present opposite viewpoints.[2] Within this new perspective, Porter addressed the history of the body, remarking that so far this had been neglected because both the classical and the Judeo-Christian traditions held a dualistic division of man, privileging mind over body. However, Porter pointed to many developments, both in academia and in society, which had stimulated greater attention for the body, also among historians: Marxism, the work of Russian philosopher and literary theorist Mikhail Bakhtin, the French Annales historians, cultural anthropology, sociology and medical sociology, feminism, historical demography, and the impact of AIDS.[3] These factors had led historians to write about, for instance, the history of pain, hysteria, sexuality, and beauty.

These new histories of the body underlined the cultural and historical variability of the body instead of viewing it as a fixed biological given. The cultural historian Thomas Laqueur, for example, argued that from antiquity to the early modern period people did not believe in the existence of two different bodies – male and female – but thought there was one type of body, of which the female was merely a less perfect version (see Chapter 4). This emphasis on the cultural history of the body was part of two, connected, innovations in history writing: the **cultural turn** and the **linguistic turn**. Although in the first half of the twentieth century some anthropologists and sociologists, as well as some of the French Annales historians, had already paid serious attention to the body, from the 1970s, and especially in the 1980s and 1990s, the cultural turn shifted the focus of research in the humanities and social sciences from socio-economic structures and events in political history to the making of meaning in daily life. This cultural turn was informed by theories from anthropology, sociology, and cultural studies. In the same period the linguistic turn, based on notions derived from philosophy and literary studies, posited that meaning is made through language, representation, and discourse. In historiography the stronger emphasis on theory resulted mostly from the impact of **poststructuralism**, which highlighted textual and discursive constructions of phenomena, and their accompanying power structures.[4]

Cultural theory was now also applied to make sense of the body as mediated through cultural sign systems. This implied a shift to *representations* of the body: rather than studying the body working, breathing, or being ill in daily life, historians now became interested in how diseases were labelled, or which body parts were believed to constitute femaleness in certain periods. Ten years after writing his 1991 article, Porter looked back upon the expansion of body history and was pleased to note that the field was booming, especially its theoretical dimension. Porter expressed dissatisfaction, however, with the theoretical approaches and methodology used by body historians. Reminding readers that body history 'is not merely a matter of crunching vital statistics, nor just a set of techniques for deciphering "representations"',[5] he warned against a one-sided reliance on theory, to the exclusion of empirical research.[6] He also noticed that much body history 'has compounded a lack of methodological sophistication with a want of scholarly rigor. Authors have sloppily conflated bodily representations with historical realities'.[7] Porter concluded that historians had neglected the ways individuals and social groups experienced their embodied selves in the past.[8]

In Porter's two review articles, the central questions in body history come to the fore: To what extent can historians reconstruct the way people in the past experienced their bodies? Can historians only approach the representation of the body in books, language, or images, or can they also gauge more individual, intimate feelings? How can they include the material aspects of the body? Should scholars study dominant prescriptions of corporeal behaviour that are imposed 'from above', by institutions or ideologies, or should they take a view 'from below', from the perspective of ordinary people? Can we then speak of bodily **'agency'**, of people's freedom to shape their own bodies? This book will review theories that have addressed these questions.

▶ The rationale behind this book

This textbook aims to provide an overview of different theoretical approaches that have been used to study the body in the past, showing how each theory highlights certain aspects of the body, and critically assessing the advantages and pitfalls of each approach. It also explores how historians uninformed by theory have – by way of their empirical research – at times come to conclusions similar to those propounded in the abstract by theorists. I am therefore careful not to depict the field of body history as solely following developments in philosophy or theory. The interactions between theory and history are manifold.

The reason why the history of the body is taken here as a separate field, even though it overlaps to some extent with other fields such as the history of medicine, **gender**, sexuality, emotion, sports, fashion, and the self, is that increasingly body history has become a specific branch of history with its own conferences and journals, and scholars identifying as body historians. The transdisciplinary journal *Body & Society*, for instance, was founded in 1995, but in practice has included more contributions from sociologists and philosophers than from historians. More recently, the German journal *Body Politics. Zeitschrift für Körpergeschichte* (founded in 2013 and including contributions in German and English) has been added to the journals publishing work on body history, though related articles can of course also be found in many other journals, mostly in those focusing on women's and gender history.

In addition to separate journals on the body, a number of multi-volume overviews of body history have been published.[9] These series, as well as a recent monograph,[10] however, pay little attention to the use of theory in body history. And while a number of textbooks have included a discussion of theoretical approaches to the body, these have mostly been written by sociologists and only include a few historical examples.[11] Therefore, this textbook aims to integrate social and cultural theory with a wealth of historical examples. In the selection of theories and histories on the body, a number of choices have been made, on the basis of my own expertise, which lies mostly in the cultural and social history of the western world in the early modern and modern periods. Ancient and medieval ideas on the body are discussed only in Chapter 1, which provides a historical overview of the most important changes in the representation of the body. Generally, the modern period is taken as point of reference. Furthermore, although this textbook does address the issues of race and (post)colonialism in several chapters, further research is needed to write a truly global history of the body.[12] Also, this book focuses mostly on cultural ideas about the body, rather than on socio-economic circumstances which impacted on people's health, and has opted to leave the interpretation of images of the body to art historians and historians of visual culture.[13]

▷ The structure of this book

After the opening chapter, which provides a historical overview of the most important continuities and changes in ideas on the body from antiquity to modernity, and explains a number of returning notions (such as **humoral theory**), the next chapters each address a body of theory and the ways historians have applied those theories. Chapter 2 discusses the influential notion of discipline, first conceptualized by sociologist Norbert Elias and philosopher Michel Foucault, as well as its corollary: bodily agency. Chapter 3 elaborates on the more general notion of social construction, including anthropological approaches such as the ideas of Mary Douglas, and theories that use the notion of the body or illness as metaphor. Chapter 4 presents the most important (feminist and queer) theories on gender and sexuality that have been formative for the field of body history, such as the work by Simone de Beauvoir, Michel Foucault, and Judith Butler. Chapter 5 focuses on a philosophical strand that is less well known among historians: that of **phenomenology**. Here, the ideas of French philosopher Maurice Merleau-Ponty are discussed, including his feminist and **postcolonial** critics (Iris Marion Young and Frantz Fanon respectively), as well as a number of historians who have used phenomenological approaches to interpret corporeal experiences in the past. Other approaches, also addressed in this chapter, which aim to zoom in on '**embodiment**' – the lived body – include Pierre

Bourdieu's notion of '**habitus**', and **psychoanalytical** analysis. Lastly, Chapter 6 reflects on the recent 'material turn' in the humanities, and its effects on theories and histories of the body. Apart from the 'neurohistorical' approach proposed by historian Daniel Lord Smail, this chapter mostly discusses '**new materialist**' scholars such as Karen Barad and Gilles Deleuze, including those new materialists who can be classified as scholars working with a **praxiographical** approach, for example Annemarie Mol.

This recent material turn in the humanities can be regarded as the second body of theories – in addition to the cultural turn – to have influenced the history of the body. This influence is still ongoing, and the impact of the material turn has not yet fully crystallized. It therefore remains to be seen what exciting new theoretical paths the history of the body will take in the future.

1 Body, Mind, and Self: Historical Perspectives

▷ Introduction

This chapter provides an overview of the main developments in the history of the human body, with the focus lying not on material changes in the body as in daily experience, or on socio-economic trends in health, poverty, and disease, but rather on cultural images of the body. Since it is impossible to be exhaustive, several choices have been made: first, I highlight important continuities, such as humoral theory, which originated in antiquity and continued to be of vital importance in making sense of the body until around 1900; second, I underline striking differences between body images in consecutive periods. Where these differences are concerned, special attention will be paid to the modern body and its relationship with the notions of mind and self.

▷ The body in antiquity and the Middle Ages

Several ideas and practices relating to the body that were established in antiquity had a long-lasting influence on the early modern and modern periods. In our modern imagination, the Olympic Games loom large; revived in 1896, they reach back as early as the eighth century BCE. These Games were known for their admiration of the male, athletic body and are seen as the start of 'the cult of the nude body as an icon of power and social rank.'[1] In the eighteenth century, influenced by recent archaeological excavations, scholars such as the German art historian and archaeologist Johann Joachim Winckelmann (1718–1768) started to define the ancient Greek statues of male bodies as models of beauty.

More influential for the view of the body from antiquity to the nineteenth century, however, was the theory of humours. Ancient authorities such as the Greek Hippocrates of Cos (c. 460–c. 370 BCE), regarded as the father of western medicine, and Galen of Pergamon (c. 130–c. 210 CE), who served as personal physician to the Roman emperor Marcus Aurelius, formulated ideas on the internal workings of the body that remained popular among doctors and laypeople until the nineteenth century. Their worldview revolved around the humours: four fluids (phlegm, black bile, yellow bile, and blood) dispersed unequally among people. Some bodies produced more black bile, giving rise to melancholy, while other bodies consisted mostly of phlegm, causing an apathetic character (the word phlegmatic stems from this humoralism). An excess or deficit of these humours was thought to lead to disease; thus the key lay in balance, to be attained via bloodletting, emetics (potions that cause vomiting), and purges.

Generally, ancient medicine was entwined with natural philosophy, sharing the subject matter of the body and its parts and fluids, including its elements of earth, air, fire, and water and its qualities such as hot, cold, wet, and dry. In the literature of classical antiquity disease was regarded as the natural condition, and health as the exception. Health could be achieved through a careful management of regimen (such as a proper diet and exercise), while disease continually threatened the body both from the outside and from within.[2]

These ideas on health and disease, in connection with humoral theory, formed the most important continuity between ancient and medieval thinking on the body. However, in the Middle Ages other views of the body were added to humoral theory. Firstly, the Middle Ages saw the elaboration of the ancient notion of the universe as a macrocosm (the heavens), and the human body as a corresponding microcosm (humans and the natural world). From the twelfth century on, medieval medicine and natural philosophy, drawing on ideas from translations of classical and Arabic texts, imagined the human body as interconnected with the stars, seasons, and elements. The moon, for example, was believed to make nails and hair grow. At least in scholarly work, the connections between microcosm and macrocosm were widespread.[3]

Secondly, the later Middle Ages brought the rediscovery of human anatomy. Dissections of human bodies had been carried out in Alexandria in the third century BCE, but the practice had been abandoned.[4] There were several motives for examining the inner parts of the body, Katharine Park claims in her study of the revival of anatomical dissection in later-medieval northern Italy. Apart from medical and forensic interests, dissection could also be prompted by spiritual motives. After the death of Chiara of Montefalco (d. 1308), for example, her fellow nuns opened up her body in search of physical signs of her saintliness. They found a crucifix in her heart and three stones in her gallbladder, which were identified with the Trinity. Park demonstrates that anatomical dissection was used not only to determine the cause of death, but also to assess disease and its possible implications for the heirs of upper-class families, with women often taking the initiative.[5]

Thirdly, the Middle Ages witnessed the growing impact of Christianity, though its precise influence on the medieval view of the body has been heavily debated. Christianity's sway over views of the body was particularly strong in relation to sexuality. Christian commentators increasingly distinguished natural from unnatural sexual activity, the former referring to reproduction. However, sex was only tolerated within the bounds of marriage, as a control for lust, while chastity was the ideal. Peter Brown has demonstrated that in Christian groups in the late Roman world, practices of sexual renunciation, continence, and celibacy were paramount.[6] Virginity, moreover, was widely recognized as a mental and spiritual condition, as well as a physical one. Consequently, medieval virginity meant the renunciation of all forms of sexual activity, including masturbation and impure thoughts.[7]

It is commonly thought that Christianity opposed a pure soul to sinful flesh. This dichotomy between body and mind could lead either to a view of the sinful body hindering the spiritual progress of Christians or to the idea of the body as a holistic unit whose coherence was guaranteed by Christian faith.[8] Historians of Christianity, however, have pointed out that the body was often seen as inseparable from the soul, for instance when martyrs used their empathic bodies to feel the presence of God and to convey his love to others, or when mystics claimed to touch and embrace God with their bodies, or even to breastfeed him or have sex with him. Christian traditions like the veneration of the wounds of Christ and of the Virgin Mary's role as a nursing mother stemmed from the Middle Ages.[9] Therefore Samantha Riches and Bettina Bildhauer state that 'many medieval religious models combined the idea of the body as earthbound and distinct from the soul with an understanding that the body could access the transcendental and was in actuality inseparable from the soul.'[10]

Similarly, Christian views on death complicate a simple body-mind dichotomy. On the one hand, in Christian theology death was seen as the moment when soul and body were separated, the soul going to heaven, hell, or purgatory, while the body rotted in the grave. Body and soul were then reunited at the Last Judgement, when the person acquired a new body. On the other hand, many people saw more continuity between life and death: the material process of cooling and drying applied not only to the living, humoral body, but also to the corpse in a tomb. It was believed that the corpse would continue to feel and move, even after burial, a belief which surfaces in the idea that the corpse of a murder victim bled when the murderer came near, thus revealing the killer.[11]

Medievalist Caroline Bynum also nuances the idea that medieval Christianity revolved around a simple body-mind **dualism**. Bynum argues that a threefold categorization was used: body (corpus), spirit (animus or spiritus), and soul (anima). Discussions in late medieval philosophy, furthermore, drew a sharper distinction between levels of soul than between soul and body.[12] Specifically, Bynum focuses on the Christian doctrine of the resurrection of the flesh, in the period between the third and fourteenth centuries. The late antique and medieval authors Bynum discusses regarded the body as a locus of eating, digestion, and excretion, and the human cadaver as a place of putrefaction. In this era, death and bodily disintegration were inextricably connected to the Christian view of the body. Since the body was changeable, constantly eating and being eaten – by worms after death for example – as well as growing and decomposing, Christian authors wondered what exactly constituted human personhood over time. Medieval theologians debated the state of the immortal body after resurrection: Would bodies that had limbs amputated during life be restored to corporeal integrity at the Day of Judgement? And what happened to cut hair, fingernails, and aborted foetuses? The doctrine of the resurrection of the flesh was, according to Bynum, formulated to reassure those afraid of the undermining of human identity by biological processes. Nevertheless, in these doctrines body and soul were not separated: the self was not associated merely with the soul. After death, body and soul were connected and together constituted the human self. The resurrected body was immortal and idealized, and at the same time grounded in individual and unique markers of sex, social status, and religious affiliation. Bynum argues that it is this medieval conception of the resurrected body as unique and intrinsic to the self that influenced modern conceptions of the relationship between body and self:

> The idea of person, bequeathed by the Middle Ages to the Modern World, was not a concept of soul escaping body, or soul using body; it was a concept of self in which physicality was integrally bound to sensation, emotion, reasoning, identity – and therefore finally to whatever one means by salvation. Despite its suspicion of flesh and lust Western Christianity did not hate or discount the body. Indeed, person was not person without the body, and body was the carrier or the expression [...] of what we today call individuality.[13]

In the High Middle Ages, so Bynum argues, a greater confidence in the relationship between the self and the physical body surfaced. The sacrament of the Eucharist, for instance, claimed that Christ's body remained whole regardless of the multiple consumption of the host by communicants. Similarly, the bodies of saints, nobles, and prelates were now seen as having a wholeness in spite of being partitioned: their body parts were distributed to different places after death because these parts would keep radiating the person's magical power. Such relics were thought to allow access to the divine and to offer protection. A saint's finger was seen to represent his full self, not just a part of his body, and saints' corpses were venerated accordingly. Bynum's work thus highlights both the magical aspects of the medieval body and corpse and those connections between body and self that point to 'modernity'. It underlines that medieval Christian thought is more complicated than the notion of body–mind dualism can allow for.

▷ The body in the early modern period

Ideas on the body in antiquity, the Middle Ages, and the early modern period show a great deal of continuity. Humoral theory continued to be the basis of interpretations of health, disease, and bodily difference. At the same time, new conceptions of the body were presented. On the one hand, these derived from discoveries by physicians and scientists. In 1543 the Flemish anatomist and physician Andreas Vesalius (1514–1564) published *On the Fabric of the Human Body*, a book based on personal observation of corpses and living bodies and partly criticizing ancient authorities such as Galen. Vesalius' magnum opus is regarded as one of the foundations of modern observational science and anatomy.[14] Other important landmarks in the history of medicine included the discovery of the system of blood circulation to the heart and brain by English physician William Harvey (1578–1657), as described in his 1628 book *On the Motion of the Heart and Blood*. Works like those written by Vesalius and Harvey marked the start of the demise of the influence of ancient medicine.[15]

On the other hand, natural philosophy also made its contribution to theorizing the body anew. Famously, philosopher René Descartes (1596–1650) privileged rational subjectivity, or the thinking being (*'Cogito ergo sum'*. 'I think therefore I am'), and separated the thinking mind from the body. This so-called **Cartesian dualism** implied that subjectivity became disembodied, and the body became regarded as a machine.[16] This turn to a new dualism of body and mind has been traced beyond philosophy and science. Jonathan Sawday argues that the Renaissance witnessed a new culture of dissection, which was strongly connected with the imaginative arts. Anatomy was not only depicted in famous paintings like Rembrandt's The Anatomy Lesson of Dr Nicolaes Tulp (1632), but also drew the attention of laypeople, who flocked to attend dissections of executed criminals. This fascination with dissection led to a new view of the body, Sawday holds. Whereas in the early Renaissance, investigation of the body could not be separated from thinking about its soul or sensibility, this idea was gradually replaced by an image of the body as a machine: 'As a machine, the body became objectified: a focus of intense curiosity, but entirely divorced from the world of the speaking and thinking object.'[17] This was a shift from giving the body spiritual meaning to a new rationalism, which focused on its usefulness, a view which had taken root by the late seventeenth century.[18]

However, it is questionable whether these new intellectual views of the mechanistic body really influenced the interactions between people of all social classes. Due to the availability of primary sources such as letters, diaries, ballads, jest books, popular medical manuals, and court records, historians have been able to minutely sketch the ways common people thought about the body.[19] Laura Gowing, for instance, has reconstructed the relationship between the body as a cultural construction and its corporeal experience in seventeenth-century England. Compared to modern ideas of the body, this period saw different body boundaries: mental and physical subjectivity were entwined, and subjectivity had a strong collective aspect, since the individual was embedded in tight social networks. Sex, pregnancy, and reproduction, particularly where women were concerned, were subjected to social control, by men but also by women, especially family members and married female neighbours.[20] Juries of matrons examined women's bodies in cases of rape, infanticide, or the non-consummation of marriage.[21] Women's chastity was vital to social order, and hence women were encouraged to be sexually passive and to keep their bodies to the private sphere. At the same time, humoral theory stressed that vaginas were active, devouring organs, and sexually voracious women required an orgasm to conceive. As Gowing concludes: 'The great power of early modern models of the body was their flexibility: alongside the process of professionalization the popular culture of the body retained its hold, and popular and official medical cultures continued to intersect.'[22]

In the Renaissance, magical beliefs still formed a strong undercurrent not only in daily life, but also in medical thought. We encounter this magic in the ideas on how to identify the body of a witch. The signs revealing the witch's body included moles, extra nipples, and insensitive body areas. It was commonly thought that the body of a witch could not be pierced by shot or by a pin, because her blood was so thick with old age, and so lacking in fire, that it could not be extracted. The hard body of the witch was the opposite of the soft body of the mother. Inexplicable wounds, bruises, or blood spots on the witch's body were seen as the devil's secret mark after the sealing of his pact with the witch. A misplaced nipple from which the devil could feed might reveal the witch's identity, again indicating a perversion of motherhood. These magical beliefs were, however, not limited to witches. It was also commonly believed that murderers could be identified by the reappearance of blood on their hands, as when – in Shakespeare's famous early seventeenth-century tragedy *Macbeth* – Lady Macbeth cannot rid herself of her victim's blood when she tries to wash it off her hands.[23] Hence, historians suggest that alongside the new Cartesian dualism and the new view of the body as machine, multiple flexible notions of the body, including the belief in the magical properties of the body, continued to exist at the level of popular belief.

▶ Colonial perspectives on race and the body

In addition to the novel conception of the body as a machine, a major shift in cultural views on the body was brought on by voyages of discovery and by colonization, which highlighted racial differences. Historians debate the origins of racial classification, variously dating it to antiquity, the Middle Ages, the early modern era, and the modern period, but they are in agreement about the importance of colonialism and slavery in accelerating the allocation of differences between human beings with different skin colours. Up to the fourteenth century, in western Europe religious and 'ethnic' variations in behaviour were far more significant than physical differences. Most distinctions were based on differences in hair and dress, rather than skin and face. Muslims, for instance, were recognized by their turbans, and Irish men by their long beards. However, the exceptions were black people, who were identified on the basis of their dark skin and accompanying facial features, and Jews, whose supposedly hooked noses were singled out to distinguish them from other people.[24]

Colonialism had a direct and devastating effect on the bodies of indigenous people in the Americas, Africa, and Australia, who were decimated by the introduction of European diseases such as measles or smallpox. In addition, bodies were central as 'sites through which imperial and colonial power was imagined and exercised'.[25] For example, sixteenth- and seventeenth-century English explorers and travel writers depicted African and Amerindian women in the new world as monstrous and inhuman, thereby justifying European colonialism. Indigenous women were portrayed as wild labouring beasts, with long hair down to their waist and sagging breasts. Their fecundity was seen to go hand in hand with their capacity for manual work, an argument used to demonstrate their capacity for hard labour.[26] It is therefore also argued by historians that slavery contributed much to the increasing importance of physical features in seventeenth- and eighteenth-century classification systems. Susan Dwyer Amussen argues that in the Caribbean from the 1660s onwards English colonial officials began to identify slavery as inherent in bodies, rather than as a product of law or a system of labour, thus prioritizing skin colour over social status in designating difference between human beings.[27] Racial difference thus became naturalized.

The voyages of discovery and the ensuing process of colonization, which brought Europeans into contact with different people, led to academic attempts at classifying human races in the eighteenth century. Scholars debated whether racial characteristics were innate or formed over a number of years by the environment, such as climate, diet, customs, and disease. The debate focused mostly on the shape of the skull, nose, and lips, on the colour of skin and texture of hair, and later on the skeleton. Physical anthropologists of the 'environmentalist' school, such as the German Johann Blumenbach (1752–1840) and the Frenchman Georges-Leclerc de Buffon (1707–1788), posited that the noses of African babies were flat because their heads pounded against their mothers' bodies during household tasks and domestic labour.[28] Eighteenth-century science thus contributed to the classification and attribution of racial variations, but its view of varieties of humankind as 'dynamic entities' was different from the solid and reified categories of nineteenth-century racial science, which was hallmarked by white supremacy.[29]

Race intersected with gender and class in these new ideas on the classification of humankind. In the discourse of the European nineteenth-century elite, the white, adult, rational, middle-class man was contrasted with other groups regarded to be closer to nature and animals: women, children, the working class, and non-white people. These contrasts were expressed in binary oppositions such as white-black, clean-dirty, respectable-nonrespectable, and pure-impure, which, moreover, played out on the body: whereas Victorian ladies covered their fair skins, working women were suntanned and bared parts of their bodies. White, delicate hands symbolized both gentility and femininity; rough hands testified to manual labour and masculinity.[30] In this way, class society was naturalized, bodily difference not being seen as a result of performing certain tasks, but as an original, inborn hallmark.

▶ The body and modernity: Science and medicine

In the nineteenth century, nature and biology took the place of religion and custom in explaining racial, class, and gender difference, and the shape and condition of bodies in general. Only then would physicians definitively distance themselves from the humoral paradigm, even though popular culture remained saturated with humoral notions of the body, disease, and character. Earlier, the theory of humours had slowly been replaced by a focus on fibres and specific organs. Increasingly, the inner body was described as a solid, compact, and closed entity.[31] In the nineteenth century, however, the body became **medicalized**, and disease concepts became increasingly anatomical. The death blow to the theory of humours was delivered by the discovery of cell theory (namely the interpretation of disease in terms of cellular alteration) by the German pathologist Rudolf Virchow (1821–1902) in 1858. Last, humoralism was swept aside by the discovery of germs – microorganisms which can cause disease – in laboratories such as that led by French (micro) biologist and chemist Louis Pasteur (1822–1895), later viewed as one of the founders of bacteriology.[32] The discovery of germs also led to the disappearance of the theory of miasma. In this theory, derived from humoralism, miasma – a kind of foul air – was long regarded as causing and transmitting diseases such as cholera and typhus. In the late nineteenth century it was replaced with a discourse on hygiene that emphasized clean water and sanitation.[33]

In addition to this transformation of the main conception of the body, the second major shift in medical theory and practice in the modern period related to a new location and manner of treatment. Even from the late seventeenth century, midwives' and married women's natural authority over the female body and reproduction had gradually been usurped by professional male doctors and male midwives.[34] In other respects, too, a process of (academic) professionalization can be seen. Until the eighteenth and nineteenth centuries, doctors mostly confined their physical examination of patients to hands, pulse, and face, or to body fluids like urine. This so-called bedside medicine focused mostly on a discussion of symptoms between doctor and patient and often resulted in the two agreeing on the diagnosis and treatment.[35] In the second half of the nineteenth century, beginning in France, a shift took place from bedside medicine to 'hospital medicine': medicine became based on pathology, and patients were treated in hospitals (often teaching hospitals).[36] The patient now submitted to the physician's authority, and the diagnosis followed from the reading of signs from the body by auscultation or percussion, rather than on the agreement between doctor and patient in regard to bodily symptoms and their treatment. Instead of prognosis and treatment, diagnosis took centre stage, and the patient became subject to the hospital regime. In the clinic, autopsies also helped physicians to gain knowledge of the body. Pain and symptoms were no longer solely pointers to the classification of diseases, but clues directing the doctor to the organs and tissues in which the illness was located, a mere guide to the underlying pathology, which provided the only reliable basis of diagnosing disease.[37] Whereas in early eighteenth-century bedside medicine the illness was the same as the pain or symptom reported by the patient (for instance headache), under the regime of hospital medicine it was ultimately the examining gaze of the physician that penetrated the body to locate the disease in particular sites in the body. As Foucault writes, the question asked to the sick patient was no longer 'what is the matter with you?', but 'where does it hurt?'.[38] This move towards an organ-orientated medicine is seen by scholars as a marginalization of the patient's voice.[39]

The third key change in medical theory and practice took place in the nineteenth century, when psychiatry evolved into a separate and new discipline. This development started from a new attention to 'nervous physiology', which traced the connections between the nerves, organs, and disease. Until the mid-nineteenth century, medicine was **'psychosomatic'**: no boundaries were perceived between doctors specializing in the body and those focused on the mind. 'Alienists', as early psychiatrists were known (a reference to diseases that alienated patients from reality), were primarily preoccupied with the definition and classification of neurosis, forging links between physical changes in the nervous system and behavioural disorders. The new academic field of psychiatry was optimistic regarding the future cure of mental patients, as is also testified by newly built asylums. Psychiatric disorders were increasingly perceived as disorders of the brain, rather than of the soul, justifying physical treatments.[40] The brain had acquired the status of most important human organ. Whereas in humoral theory the heart was regarded as the centre of emotions, capturing the essence of humanity,[41] in the nineteenth century the brain came to occupy central stage, replacing the concept of the soul, a regime Fernando Vidal has termed 'brainhood'.[42]

The new psychiatric authority in relation to matters of the mind also comes to the fore in the modern notion of (psychological) 'trauma'. The term, coined in the 1870s by psychiatrists who applied it to the psychological consequences of railway accidents, connected physical hurt with recurring mental effects.[43] Later, the similar concept of 'shell shock' was applied to the traumatic experiences of soldiers during the First World War.[44] The new concept of trauma can also be traced in the medical discussion on the effects of sexual violence. In the vocabulary of humours, which had a lasting influence until the late nineteenth century, the mind was inextricably connected to the body. In rape cases, for instance, the traumatic experience of victims was hardly addressed: attention was mostly directed to traces of violence on the body. Doctors noted the impact of rape on morals, especially the loss of virginity or the risk of corruption, but never referred to structural mental effects. Those effects were not completely denied, but were rather described in terms of 'fright'. For example, it was very common for girls and women to refer to their menstruation suddenly having stopped after a shocking sight or experience. In this perspective, mind and body were aligned.[45] It is especially from psychoanalysis that we know the idea of mental trauma as a result of sexual violation, which, however, would only become widespread later in the twentieth century.[46]

In addition to the professionalization of medicine and the rise of psychiatry, the nineteenth century saw the emergence of new perspectives on the body, both academic and popular. One such perspective, **phrenology**, built on a much older tradition of analyzing character on the basis of facial features. Even in ancient Greece, texts theorized about the notion of inner character being reflected in looks, and in bodily features such as the face, head, hair, and skin.

In the later Middle Ages, attention turned to the significance of the appearance of the genitalia, and to the female body. It was held, for instance, that the size of a man's nose correlated with the size of his penis.[47] This tradition was revived in the eighteenth and nineteenth centuries, first by the theologian, writer, and philosopher Johann Kasper Lavater (1741–1801) who developed **physiognomy**, the 'science' of reading the shape of faces. Thus, intelligence could be read from the forehead, moral feeling and sensibility from the surface between the eyebrows and the lower lip, and sensuality from the neck. Silhouette portraits gained popularity as instruments for a physiognomic examination.[48] Similarly, phrenology was later developed in 1796 by the German physician Franz Joseph Gall (1758–1828). Phrenologists claimed that the human mind was composed of various mental faculties in conjunction. Each particular faculty was found in a corresponding area in the brain. In practice the head could be examined by searching for bumps, which were regarded as places where the brain showed strong activity. The 'organs' of Destructiveness and Secretiveness, for instance, were to be found in the area of the skull just above the ears. Phrenology offered a way of getting to know a person's character by studying the face and the skull.[49] It therefore represented an early kind of what Joseph Dumit calls 'objective self-fashioning': under the influence of popular knowledge of human-related sciences, the self could be made with the help of facts regarding the body and the brain, provided by science and medicine.[50]

Whereas phrenology would soon be regarded as a pseudo-science, other new ways of measuring the body came to form the basis of modern biometrics. One such example is the anthropometric system designed in the late nineteenth century by the French scientist and police officer Alphonse Bertillon (1853–1914): it was used to measure several body parts of criminals, who were also photographed, and the measurements were noted down on special forms. Its goal – to identify recidivist criminals – was not attained, since the forms were not efficiently archived and the system was abolished in the first decade of the twentieth century. The underlying idea lived on, however, in the more successful technology of fingerprinting, introduced in the 1890s. Simon Cole argues that the new use of fingerprints has led to identity being reduced to biology and demonstrated with hard scientific evidence.[51]

However, this scientific focus on measurement often went hand in hand with older pseudo-scientific ideas, building on physiognomy and phrenology. The Italian criminal anthropologist Cesare Lombroso (1835–1909), for instance, combined quantifying techniques with theories on **degeneration** – a concept from the nineteenth-century social and biological sciences referring to the deterioration of the race, attested by the 'inferior' looks and bodies of the lower classes and non-white people. Lombroso argued that the 'born criminal' could be anatomically identified by, among other features, a sloping forehead, unusually large ears, facial asymmetry, excessively long arms, cranial asymmetry, and thick, interconnected eyebrows.[52]

▶ The modern self

In addition to objective self-fashioning, carried out using body technologies such as phrenology and biometrics, historians have also analyzed how the modern self was fashioned more subjectively: the new, modern phenomenon of personal, inner, identity. Philosophers and intellectual historians have traced a progression, in texts by famous philosophers and authors, from conventional, collective, and religious societies to modern ideas of the autonomous, whole, and authentic individual.[53] Using cultural texts written for larger audiences, the cultural historian Dror Wahrman has argued that a modern regime of selfhood took root around 1780. No longer was identity seen as a group membership, which could easily be exchanged for another; on the contrary, the individual modern self came to be characterized by 'psychological depth, or interiority', and viewed as innate, natural, and unchanging. Whereas in the eighteenth century women could easily dress up in men's clothes, for example, and vice versa, in the nineteenth century male and female dress were strictly separated. Gender, moreover, came to refer to a natural, fixed identity. The same applied to identity categories like race. Wahrman posits that in the eighteenth century people thought that racial identity depended on the country one lived in, and could thus be changed by travelling. A black African would grow to be white if he lived in England. But in the nineteenth century, race and skin colour acquired their naturalistic and innate connotations that have become so familiar from histories of racism.

This new sense of self can also be discerned in portrait painting, which in the middle of the eighteenth century aimed not at capturing the individual likeness and personality of the sitter, but rather at depicting him or her as a general 'type' of character, by focusing on dress and accessories. These indicated surface appearance and cultural references, not the inner, unique self as evidenced by individual facial features. Many sitters also dressed up in masquerade, whose identity-bending options enjoyed wide popularity, until it fell into disrepute around 1800, which for Wahrman is evidence for the rise of the modern regime of self.[54]

Although the origin of this modern regime of self is unclear, there generally seems to be a consensus among historians about the novelty of modern selfhood. However, exactly when, where and how this development can be situated is still an open question. We have already seen that the medievalist Bynum regards the medieval connection between self and body as a precursor to modern notions of individuality. Despite the debate on the concept's chronological origins, it is clear that modern identity was and is inextricably connected to the body as a slate upon which to display this self.

One area in which we can identify a shift towards a modern self with bodily integrity is the cultural views of the rape of women. In the Middle Ages and early modern period rape was regarded as a property offence, since women's bodies were seen to belong to their fathers or husbands. Increasingly, however, the self of the victim was accentuated. Early modernists have argued that from the late sixteenth century rape came to be seen as a crime against an individual woman's body rather than against male property.[55] Similarly, from the nineteenth century onwards issues like free will and the possibility of consent were discussed among legal scholars and doctors. During this period, support grew for the view that a victim could be forced into sexual intercourse by mental threats, rather than by physical violence.[56] Generally, the history of rape shows that a modern, individual identity encompasses bodily integrity and self-possession.

This modern notion of individual identity has also been noted by scholars of masculinity. George L. Mosse demonstrates that the modern male body needs to be shaped and disciplined. Focusing especially on Germany, Mosse argues that modern masculinity originated in western Europe between the second half of the eighteenth century and the beginning of the nineteenth. The body became the chief signifier of manliness. The model for the ideal male body was found in the ancient Greek ideal of the beauty of harmony, control, and proportion, with an emphasis on dynamic virility. Physical beauty was an indicator of strong willpower, moral fortitude, and martial nobility. Gymnastics and athletics were the means to achieve this masculine body and self. In the nineteenth century, the modern ideal of masculinity was infused with nationalism. It was this male body that was later also celebrated in fascist movements.[57] Again we see here how the modern (male) body is based on a bodily self, but at the same time needed to be shaped according to ideals (whether personal or national).

Other historians have shown how twentieth-century women also used gymnastics to shape an active, healthy body and thus built their modern selves on sporty bodies. As Charlotte Macdonald argues, female agency can be found in women's exercise of their bodies, for example in the Women's League for Health and Beauty, founded in Britain in 1930. The League staged its large-scale demonstrations, at which hundreds of women, dressed in sleeveless white shirts and black satin shorts or velvet skirts, performed choreographed exercises and dance routines before live audiences and moving cameras at London's Hyde Park and the Royal Albert Hall.[58] The modern notion of the active body connected the body with fitness and health and, Macdonald argues, allowed women to develop a 'modern self', in which body, mind, and self were inextricably connected: 'The interwar language of health and beauty was itself a language of the self'.[59] Thus, the modern body was not only connected to individual character, but also needed 'work'.

▶ The slim body as modern body?

The emphasis on the shaping of the modern bodily self clearly comes to the fore where body size is concerned. Though fat people were not universally revered in pre-modern times, as some historians have claimed, the appreciation of oversized bodies has nevertheless been subject to historical change.[60] Between 1860 and 1920 fat came no longer to be seen as a symbol of wealth, but as a symbol of immobility and self-indulgence. Historians differ in their explanations of this shift, however. Some scholars point to the new modern guiding principles of science, and the idea of a struggle for the survival of the fittest. New nutritional knowledge provided input for seeing the body as a barometer of evolutionary fitness. Techniques such as mapping out height–weight charts and counting calories served to measure and classify human bodies. The idea of a successful self came to be connected to having a fit body of the right size and weight. A fit body was seen as key to becoming an enlightened citizen, endowed with self-control and willpower. Fatness was now associated with self-indulgence, the antithesis of liberal citizenship.[61] Other factors that played a role were the medical establishment and the insurance industry, which advocated a thinner body for reasons of health and financial gain, respectively.[62] Furthermore, Chris Forth argues that the new aversion to fat can be related to a denigration of fat as filth, which was now associated with lower-class and non-white people, an aversion stimulated by tales of European exploration and colonization. Forth points to a heightened distaste for human animality and organicity, which clashed with a self-image of white personal hygiene.[63] Fat, in short, became an 'alien invader of the civilized white body'.[64]

In addition to a class and racial dimension, the new ideals of slimness were also gendered. The impact of these for women, however, are debated among historians. Stearns argues that the idea that fat is bad predates new women's fashions or commercial appeals. He points rather to the insistence on self-control, a corollary to new areas of greater freedom: disciplined eating was a moral tool in a society where growing consumerism and more abundant leisure time seemed to contradict the work ethic of the middle class.[65] Nevertheless Stearns, and other historians, also regard the attack on women's weight in the 1920s – focusing on their physical frailty and slenderness – as a response to women's growing power in the public sphere (see Chapter 2).[66] In any case, what is certain is that the new emphasis on slimness dovetails with the sculpture that needs to be done in order for the modern body to attain the right shape.

▶ Conclusion

The history of the body – to the extent to which it has been uncovered by historians – shows several continuities. Humoral theory, for instance, was of vital importance from antiquity until the beginning of the modern era, and many humoral notions continue to live on in metaphors and sayings. Throughout history, people have scrutinized faces, from physiognomy to modern biometrics. Major shifts in conceptualizing the body were brought on the heels of Christianity, which emphasized the duality between spiritual mind, and the lowlier, fleshy body, although historians have recently argued that this duality was less strict than is often assumed. A second wave of change in ideas about the body accompanied the scientific discoveries of the seventeenth century. The body slowly came to be regarded as a machine, and this notion also contributed to the separation of mind and body. During the age of industrialization the productivity of the body as machine would be emphasized. Lastly, modernity can be seen to have witnessed a novel type of body, caused by discoveries made by medical science, focusing on cell theory, germs, and solid organs; moreover, this particular medical practice took place in academic hospitals and laboratories. New ideals of slimness and health also played their part. The emphasis on a modern, inner, and unique self required a fit body, and thus self-discipline. In Chapter 2, therefore, we will analyze how historians and other scholars have theorized the disciplined body.

2 The Modern Body, Discipline, and Agency

▶ Introduction

The first books on the history of the body often started from the premise that bodies in the past were disciplined. This chapter discusses the two most prominent theoretical perspectives on corporeal discipline: that of Norbert Elias on the civilizing process, and that of Michel Foucault on docile bodies. It furthermore addresses postcolonial critiques on the notion of 'civilization' and the role of the body in these critiques.

This chapter also shows how historians of the body have used these theoretical approaches. Specifically, the history of beauty practices is discussed to show the tension between, on the one hand, approaches that emphasize the disciplining of the body, and, on the other, those that stress individual agency (the leeway to act and make decisions). The discussions on discipline and agency strongly influenced historical debate in the final decades of the twentieth century. The last part of the chapter is devoted to body politics: political movements such as second-wave feminism, the civil rights movements, the disability rights movement, and the fat acceptance movement, all of which advocate body ownership.

▶ Elias and the civilizing process

The first scholar to write a long-term history of bodily restraint was the German sociologist Norbert Elias (1897–1990). In his book *The Civilizing Process*, originally published in German in 1939, but not available in English translation until 1978, Elias traces a shift in behaviour in western Europe: from the Middle

Ages, characterized by the unrestrained expression of emotion, and a lack of manners and privacy, to the modern period, in which composed and refined bodily behaviour was the ideal. In this view, medieval men and women were accustomed to (unpredictable) violence, torture, and killing in daily life, and did not hold back their emotions or sexual urges. By contrast, from the early modern period onwards, starting at the absolutist courts, table manners, emotional restraint, and the proper corporeal stance became highly important to the elite, and they later trickled down to the lower classes. Giving in to impulsive behaviour made way for the rationality of long-term planning. Crucially, these new behavioural codes were initially imposed by the state, but slowly were internalized by individuals. Using etiquette books as source, Elias points out major changes in the view of the body, such as the growing disgust regarding bodily waste, the disappearance of spitting in public, and the increasing use of handkerchiefs to blow one's nose.

These changes were all part of a new emphasis on privacy, which was also attested by the building of houses with private bedrooms and toilets. No longer was it customary to share a bed with visitors or servants or to perform bodily functions before others. Whereas in medieval society it was quite normal to sleep naked, this lack of inhibition disappeared rapidly in the seventeenth, eighteenth, and nineteenth centuries, as is discernible for instance in the use of designated nightwear, which Elias characterizes, like the fork and the handkerchief, as a 'tool of civilization'.[1] In his focus on inhibition and shame, Elias was influenced by Sigmund Freud's idea of the super-ego as a constraining consciousness, the internalization of the rule of the father. Freud's study *Das Unbehagen in der Kultur* (*Civilization and its Discontents*, 1930) had depicted civilization as a process in which human beings had built a functioning society, including wonderful features of art and science, but at the cost of repressing their lusts and instincts.

Elias accounts for these changes by pointing to structural processes such as the state's acquisition of monopolies on violence – banishing the random use of violence in public – and on tax collection. The German sociologist accords a pivotal role to the court societies of France, England, and Germany. Whereas the medieval knight was free to express emotions and use violence as he pleased, the court nobility in the seventeenth and eighteenth centuries became dependent on the king, who prescribed diplomacy and restraint, and who had taken away the knights' traditional role as warriors. At court, elaborate rules of conduct developed, which the nobility could use to find favour with the king, but also to distinguish themselves from groups like the bourgeoisie. Strong social control intensified, and speech, posture, and appearance were minutely inspected:

> To keep one's place in the intense competition for importance at court, to avoid being exposed to scorn, contempt, loss of prestige, one must subordinate one's appearance and gestures, in short oneself, to the fluctuating norms of court society that increasingly emphasize the difference, the distinction of the people belonging to it. One *must* wear certain materials and certain shoes. One *must* move in certain ways characteristic of people belonging to court society. Even smiling is shaped by court custom.[2]

Generally, people grew mutually dependent and thus increasingly had to take account of each other. This new scrutiny of behaviour led to greater identification between people. Fears of attack were replaced by social fears of shame and embarrassment.[3] The creation of these 'civilized bodies' involved, as sociologist Chris Shilling notes, 'a progressive socialization, rationalization and individualization of the body.'[4]

The strength of Elias' work lies in its combination of diverse social processes over a longer period of time. In all these processes – the transformation in affect control, the restraint of violence, and the webs of interdependence – the body assumes a central position. As Shilling argues, Elias outlines the relationships between embodied subjects: subjects whose bodies are connected with their minds, capacities, and desires, and who respond to other embodied subjects. Elias thus moves beyond a simple notion of the body to the notion of embodiment.[5] In this way, he demonstrates how the body is both socially constructed and at the same time a natural entity.[6] Bodies develop in a social context and in relation to other bodies (in 'social figurations'). For Elias the civilizing process is an evolutionary process, which accentuates the body's increasing socialization at the cost of biological urges and desires.[7]

criticism

The Civilizing Process has been criticized by medievalists, who perhaps understandably did not agree with Elias' image of the medieval lack of restraint.[8] In addition, scholars have argued that the concept of civilization might be too undifferentiated to account for paradoxical developments: as Shilling notes, contemporary capitalism might force employees to discipline themselves at work, but the home or other places of relaxation might demonstrate individuals' selective application of these disciplinary norms.[9] Thirdly, it has been commented that the civilizing process seems to be an anonymous process, leaving little room for conscious, individual agency.[10] Fourthly, historians have been critical of Elias' use of etiquette books. For him, these straightforwardly reflected the 'affective structure' of a group; however, critics have pointed out that the relationship between the prescriptive nature of these texts and the social reality might be more complex.[11]

Despite these criticisms, however, the notion of the civilizing process in general has been accepted by many scholars and has influenced research on, for instance, the history of sport. Elias himself put forward the view that with the banishment of violence and excitement in modern civilization, sport emerged as a relatively non-violent form of physical contest, a way in which excitement could still be channelled.[12] Boxing, for example, became a tamed and regulated channelling of men's aggression, including the wearing of padded gloves, just as duelling provided an outlet for the aristocracy.[13]

The notion of the civilizing process has also impacted the history of emotions. Historian Barbara Rosenwein, for example, appreciates the room Elias' theory makes for change, its provision of explanations for this change, and the space it accords to emotion. However, she dismisses the hydraulic model of emotions applied by Elias and Freud, in which universal emotions are either 'on' or 'off', depending on their repression by society, the individual, or the super-ego, and are always searching for an outlet. Rosenwein prefers a **social constructionist** approach to emotions, since every culture has rules about emotions and thus emotional restraints, which change over time. For Rosenwein, Elias did not take sufficient account of the cultural and emotional communities involved.[14]

Despite these points of critique, Elias' concept of the civilizing process still carries much weight in historical and sociological scholarship. It was one of the earliest theories that took the body seriously. Later in the twentieth century, a renewed emphasis on the disciplined body would feature in the work of, most importantly, Foucault.

▶ The body and modern discipline: Foucault

This discipline which according to Elias was a hallmark of the civilizing process has featured in other theories in slightly different ways. In 1967, the British labour historian E.P. Thompson (1924–1993) already remarked on industrial capitalism's enforcement of time discipline, by clocks, bells, and fines, money incentives, preaching and schooling, the division and supervision of labour in factories, and the suppression of fairs and sports.[15] A comparable theory that has had more impact, however, is Foucault's (1926–1984) notion of modern disciplinary power, which can primarily be found in his book *Discipline and Punish. The Birth of the Prison* (1977). This book traces the changes in the practices of criminal punishment in the late eighteenth and early nineteenth centuries, which included the abolition of torture and public executions, a new focus on disciplinary incarceration in prisons, and the involvement in criminal proceedings of specialists on the criminal mind, such as forensic psychiatrists. Rather than explaining the abolition of corporeal punishment and the rise of modern discipline as an indication of humanitarian progress, Foucault is concerned with this new function of disciplinary power, which works much more invisibly than the explicit use of power by kings, politicians, or the judiciary in the early modern period.

In the new Panopticon model of the prison – the metaphor of modern disciplinary power – prisoners could be watched by guards at any time, yet never knew when they were actually being checked. Thus, prisoners disciplined their behaviour themselves, which was efficient for prison management. Foucault argues that this new disciplinary technology of power was productive, for example because more work was done efficiently by a disciplined labour force, but also because at the same time the new forensic psychiatrists and social workers enhanced the knowledge concerning human beings: 'the body becomes a useful force only if it is both a productive body and a subjected body'.[16]

Instigated by capitalism, this focus on disciplined bodies can be found not only in prisons, but also in schools and hospitals. As we saw in the previous chapter, Foucault traced the rise of the modern hospital, in which bodies become objects scrutinized by doctors who, relying on knowledge from anatomy and pathology, inspect, touch, and observe the patient's body. This expert clinical gaze involved the classification of patients' bodies, who were now gathered in one space, that of the hospital ward. Corpses were opened up and inspected in hospital mortuaries.

At the level of the state we can see this new emphasis on the classification of bodies in what Foucault called **'biopolitics'**: the state's government of its population by regulating public health, sexuality, and disease. With the help of statistics, such as birth and death rates, the modern state tried to survey and control the size and health of its residents. Examples include the state's efforts to improve public hygiene by constructing sewers and combatting infectious disease from the nineteenth century onwards, as well as twentieth-century eugenicist policies, which aimed at 'improving' a white, fit, elitist race by discouraging the reproduction of 'inferior' citizens.[17] In short, for Foucault modern discipline was a form of power found at different societal institutions.

Foucault's notion of 'docile bodies', which 'may be subjected, used, transformed and improved',[18] has been applied by other scholars. Feminist philosopher Susan Bordo argues that both in Victorian conduct manuals and in

contemporary advertisements for food, elite women were advised against indul-
gent eating and instructed how to eat in a feminine way: as little as possible,
only individually wrapped pieces of tiny, bite-size candies, and without showing
any desire.[19] Bordo concludes: 'the social control of female hunger operates as
a practical "discipline" (to use Foucault's term) that trains female bodies in the
knowledge of their limits and possibilities'.[20] Bordo also analyzes the practices
of dieting and exercise as normalizing technologies, 'insuring the production
of self-monitoring and self-disciplining "docile bodies"'.[21] Like Foucault, Bordo
here uses a notion of power that entails self-inspection, rather than an external
agent, as well as productivity.

The Foucauldian concept of disciplined, docile bodies has been interpreted in a
variety of ways. Historians have criticized Foucault's dating of the rise of modern
penal systems and their accompanying methods of disciplinary punishment.[22]
More interesting, however, are their interpretations of the role of the body in
this development. Many scholars have noted that Foucault's account of passive
bodies lacks agency, subjectivity, and experience. Some have even accused him
of 'anti-humanism'.[23] In this reading, Foucault, especially in his earlier works
such as *Discipline and Punish*, only regards bodies as produced and manipulated
by power.[24] However, other authors have pointed out that Foucault's notion of
power is much more open than a simple focus on oppression, leaving room for
contestation. Moreover, some (feminist) scholars emphasize rather that Foucault
identifies the body as a site of power, pointing to the 'local and intimate operations of power rather than focussing exclusively on the supreme power of the
state'.[25] Especially in his later work (the later volumes of his *History of Sexuality*
and his unpublished lectures), Foucault turns to the notion of '**technologies of
the self**', leaving more room for individual agency.[26] He defines technologies
of the self as permitting 'individuals to effect by their own means or with the
help of others a certain number of operations on their own bodies and souls,
thoughts, conduct, and way of being, so as to transform themselves in order to
attain a certain state of happiness, purity, wisdom, perfection, or immortality'.[27]
Here, Foucault presumes that the subject constitutes itself, by 'working on' her
body and mind, for example through self-knowledge. His notion of technologies
of the self has, however, been used by cultural historians less often than his ideas
on discipline.

One example of the way historians have discussed the concepts of discipline and
agency within the penal setting sketched by Foucault concerns the use of tattoos
by Irish prisoners in the late nineteenth century. In this period, several methods

were designed to identify prisoners in order to trace repeat offenders. Prisoners' bodily features were described in records, and from the late nineteenth century they were also photographed. To have their picture taken, Irish prisoners were positioned with their hands crossed in front of their chest, and thus 'subjected' to penal power. However, the notion of discipline does not sufficiently cover the treatment of prisoners' bodies. Interestingly, historians Ciara Breathnach and Elaine Farrell discovered that prison officials concealed tattoos using powder and paste, probably to increase uniformity. This might indicate that the tattoos on the prisoners' bodies were regarded as rebellious, possibly conveying the meaning that these prisoners were hardened by pain, or were members of a subgroup. Tattoos were most often found on hands and forearms, and frequently consisted of names, often of relatives, and numbers or maritime symbols.[28] These historians have thus found evidence of bodily agency within the prison system, but do not doubt that the disciplining of prisoners' bodies is of central importance.

To conclude: Both Elias' notion of the civilizing process and Foucault's focus on modern discipline highlight the restraining effects of social norms on bodies, and the role of self-discipline. Whereas Elias pays attention to the body as subjective agent, Foucault is more interested in outlining the discourses and practices that impact on the body as object. As Lois McNay writes, in Foucault's work '[t]here is a tendency to conceive of the body as essentially a passive, blank surface upon which power relations are inscribed'.[29] Foucault's work has also been criticized for obscuring the materiality of the body. We will return to the questions of the agency of the body in these theories later in this chapter.

▶ Postcolonial critique of 'civilized bodies'

In Elias' work, the notion of civilization may indicate bodily restraint, but nevertheless still retains its traditionally positive connotations. In recent years, however, numerous postcolonial studies have strongly criticized this western concept, which in their view was used by European colonizers to justify the latter's violent rule over 'barbaric' Others.[30] These critics argue that Elias' idea of the civilizing process ignores the violence done in the name of 'civilization', especially to non-western people.[31] Even within Europe, the Irish were long portrayed by the British as uncivilized and in need of British rule and discipline. Especially in the later nineteenth century, under the influence of Darwinism, Irish men and women were caricatured in satirical magazines with simian features, indicating that they were presumed to be closer to the ape than to the white human. But already much earlier, from the first waves of colonization in the twelfth century, English overseers described the Irish as animals: early seventeenth-century sources mentioned that the Irish diet and table manners were considered barbarous, that Irish men were condemned for wearing their hair fringes long over their eyes and Irish women for riding side-saddle the opposite way from the English.[32] Bodily features and habits were thus indicators of the lack of civilization. Emotion, too, functioned as a barometer of civilization, emotional control being regarded as a sign of cultivation, and a susceptibility to violent passions as an indicator of a lack thereof.[33]

Gender, class, and race are inextricably connected to the notion of civilization. In the nineteenth century, under the influence of theories on evolution, medical writers began to discuss the influence of the environment on gender differences, and the relationship between nature and nurture. They regarded women, children, and primitive people as stuck at an arrested stage of development of the human species.[34] Historian Laura Briggs has shown how American nineteenth-century medical and gynaecological discourse was suffused with the notion of 'civilization'. In this discourse cultural evolution had progressed from a 'barbarian' or 'savage' stage to a civilized one, although some people had either been left behind or might revert to the lower stages: the degenerate ones. Hysteria and nervousness were considered conditions of 'overcivilized' women, that is, white and upper-class women. Since frail, hysterical women were often seen as having problems with regard to sexuality and reproduction, Briggs argues that the gendered discourse on hysteria in fact overlies a discourse on race: white 'hysterical' women of the middle and upper classes were seen to endanger their kind by their infertility, whereas 'savage' people – indigenous, non-white and/or poor men and women – produced more children. Moreover, the discourse of nervousness relied on this racial theory of the existence of two different kinds of bodies: 'one white, nervous, and plagued by weakness; the other racialized, colonized, and hardy'.[35] Since black and poor women were thought to have 'underdeveloped' nervous systems, they were regarded as being unable to feel pain. As a result, nineteenth-century American gynaecologists experimented on African-American and poor women, for instance by removing their ovaries without anaesthetic.[36] Thus, the nineteenth-century discourse on civilization shows how gender, class, and race intersect in the view of bodies.

This postcolonial critique of the concept of civilization does not always, however, relate specifically to the work of Elias and Foucault. When Rao and Pierce state that '[c]orporeal techniques (torture, flogging, bodily violence) indexed, enforced, and helped to constitute categories of difference in colonial and post-colonial contexts',[37] there is no allusion to the emphasis on productivity and the lack of explicit corporeal violence as central elements of Foucault's notion of discipline. Nevertheless, much work has been done on the ways docile bodies and individuals were produced in the non-western world. A prime example is the practice of the binding of upper-class Chinese women's feet. Foot binding originated during the rule of the Song dynasty (960–1279), as a symbol of beauty but also as a sign of wealth, since small feet were associated with sexuality and maternity rather than with labouring. As revisionist history has shown, it was a practice executed by mothers on the feet of their daughters and upheld by these women, rather than by men.[38] During the late nineteenth and early twentieth centuries, anti-footbinding campaigns, instigated by the English missionary Reverend MacGowan in 1875 under the slogan 'heavenly feet', tried to eradicate this practice. As Dorothy Ko argues, these campaigns were based on the foreign construct of a God-given natural body that realizes its beauty in motion. Apart from western missionaries and a minority of educated Chinese women, it was mostly male Chinese reformers who championed the cause of anti-footbinding as part of their nationalist agenda of freeing China from the shame of backwardness. In presenting themselves as rescuers, they portrayed Chinese women with bound feet as victims.[39] In this particular history writing, less emphasis is put on the ways Chinese women's bodies were disciplined in the act of footbinding, than on the way the colonizers imposed western morality on the Chinese reformers and enforced anti-footbinding measures.[40] In the context of colonial India, the postcolonial critic Gayatri Spivak has termed this sort of appropriation of the gendered body in light of the civilizing mission as '[w]hite men are saving brown women from brown men'.[41] In this perspective, the body becomes a terrain over which colonial power relations are fought. Postcolonial analyses have thus demonstrated the exclusionary practices accompanying the notion of civilization.

▶ Beauty, discipline, and agency

One field in which bodily discipline, and its relationship to agency, occupies a prime position is the history of beauty practices and fashion. The tension between bodily discipline and agency in historical research is exemplified by the 'corset controversy'. Many historians have considered the nineteenth-century female corset as the paradigm of discipline and women's oppression. The restrictive dress of Victorian upper-class women is said to symbolize the woman's subordinate position and to limit her freedom of movement. Other scholars, however, point out that women could experience pleasure by tight-lacing their corsets, at the same time using their appearance and sexuality to climb the social ladder.[42] In this latter view Victorian women are attributed more agency.

The debate between scholars who foreground the role of discipline and those who emphasize agency also surfaces in histories of beauty practices. Historians of beauty have demonstrated the novelty of modern ideals of beauty. The American historian Joan Jacobs Brumberg, for instance, notes a shift in American beauty ideals: whereas in the nineteenth century, beauty was seen to derive from internal qualities such as moral character, spirituality, and health, in the twentieth century girls became concerned with the shape and appearance of their bodies as a primary expression of their individual identity.[43] This shift was accelerated in the late 1880s by the widespread adoption by the American middle classes of a bathroom basin with running water, and a mirror hung above it, the mirror facilitating constant facial and body inspection. But 'cultural mirrors' too, such as films and photos in magazines, led to a focus on the 'visual rather than the spiritual self'.[44] This started with the voluptuous Victorian hourglass figure, with its tiny waist and exaggerated hips:

> By the 1920s both fashion and film had encouraged a massive 'unveiling' of the female body, which meant that certain body parts – such as arms and legs – were bared and displayed in ways they had never been before. This new freedom to display the body was accompanied, however, by demanding beauty and dietary regimens that involved money as well as self-discipline. Beginning in the 1920s, women's legs and underarms had to be smooth and free of body hair; the torso had to be svelte; and the breasts were supposed to be small and firm. What American women did not realize at the time was that their stunning new freedom actually implied the need for greater internal control of the body, an imperative that would intensify and become even more powerful by the end of the twentieth century.[45]

The self-discipline surfaced for example with regard to the skin. In views on skin conditions such as acne the emphasis shifted from inner to outer qualities. Whereas in the nineteenth century adolescent acne was regarded as a sign of moral perversity (often indicating masturbation), in the early twentieth century it was seen as a marker of dirtiness and low social class. The ideas on germs, launched in the late 1870s and 1880s, led to a new awareness of dirt and squalor as generators of disease, and hence to increased hygiene for middle-class homes, bodies, and faces. In the twentieth century, perfect skin became an indicator of social success, and parents assisted their daughters with the improvement of their bodies. Each adolescent (and this held particularly for girls) was now personally responsible for maintaining proper habits of hygiene and self-discipline.[46] Thus, Brumberg speaks about the 'body project', underlining especially female adolescents' bodily self-discipline in line with cultural discourses on the svelte and clean female body.

In her study on modern German beauty practices, historian Annelie Ramsbrock also emphasizes discipline (and self-discipline) and **normalization**. From the Enlightenment, new 'natural' beauty practices became interwoven with science, for instance in the new science of dermatology, in prescriptions on bathing, washing, walking, diet, and skin cream. Scientists warned against the harmful ingredients – such as lead and mercury – of older forms of makeup, and applied new scientific inventions, for example X-rays, to cure eczema or acne. Through measurements, plastic surgeons provided an objective norm of beauty. As early as the start of the nineteenth century German surgeons performed corrective surgery on people who had lost their noses because of syphilis or a rapier duel. Yet Ramsbrock argues that these patients themselves determined that they could not live without a nose because of the strong social stigma. They clearly did not lack agency. The same applies to the new use of cosmetics and makeup by German women from the 1920s, influenced by the new consumption cultures in department stores, women's magazines, and beauty salons. Youthful and natural looks became increasingly important, also on the labour market. 'Natural', however, did not refer to nature, but to an ideal that women could attain through self-discipline. The discipline and normalization of bodies therefore was accompanied by a presentation of self that helped women and men to improve their socio-economic position. For this reason Ramsbrock also uses the Foucauldian notion of technologies of the self to indicate that makeup and cosmetics were a means that served people to work on themselves.[47] This notion here navigates between discipline and agency.

Similarly, historian Rebecca Herzig employs the concept of 'practices of the self' in her study on the history of hair removal in the United States. She notes how in the first decades of the twentieth century, women's body hair was increasingly denigrated as abnormal and dirty. Already in the nineteenth century scientists and doctors had associated abundant facial and body hair with illness and madness.

But from around 1920, American women themselves also became convinced that they had to epilate their armpits, legs, and face. Herzig points to several explanatory factors, such as the increasing importance of hygiene, novel fashions that left the lower legs and underarms bare, the new privacy offered by the arrival of bathrooms, and newly available techniques for removing hair, varying from the Gillette razor (1903) to the use of electrolysis and X-rays later in the twentieth century. Some scholars interpret the new focus on female hair removal as a form of discipline and a backlash to the new, independent role of working women, in short as an attempt to infantilize them. In this view, female body hair was taken to be a sign of manliness, and connected to women's claim to voting rights and their push for access to jobs and education: 'Visible body hair, like women's smoking, drinking, and paid labor outside the home, became a ready mark of the new woman's "excessive" sexual, political and economic independence.'[48] Herzig herself prefers to speak of 'self-discipline', since these practices of hair removal were not imposed from above, but were taken up by women themselves. At the same time, Herzig criticizes the later twentieth-century emphasis on individual freedom and the choice to take care of one's own body in beauty practices, since it obscures the influence of beauty norms and, in neoliberal fashion, masks consumption practices as individual freedom. Following Foucault, Herzig regards hair removal practices as practices of normalization, which emphasize the inner management of conduct and internal discipline. These efforts at personal transformation are, Herzig states, in fact the vessels of modern power.[49] Herzig thus follows Foucault in emphasizing self-discipline as a practice to shape the body, in which normalizing discourses are taken up by individuals who see their practices as expressions of individual freedom and care of the self.

We have seen that the issues of self-discipline and agency come to the fore especially in historical research into modern health and beauty practices. Whereas Foucault emphasized penal practice as a model for modern discipline, historians have located discipline in the daily care of the body. The early twentieth century in particular witnessed a strong emphasis on self-control, appearance, and dieting. Historian Peter Stearns therefore regards these new slenderness standards as an extension of the process of bodily discipline as described by Elias. Stearns suggests that the novel attention to weight around 1900 may have been a means for the upper classes to distinguish themselves as restrained people from the lower classes. Whereas Elias focused on bodily movements as a means of distinction, this process of discipline around 1900 began to relate to the shape and appearance of the body.[50] Self-discipline and social distinction are again connected in the manner suggested by Elias.

▶ Body politics

In the scholarly discussions of modern disciplining practices, discipline is often contrasted with agency. The notion of agency, however, is more complex than it might seem. In the following section I discuss the 'body politics' which played such a central role in second-wave feminism and the movements for civil rights, disability rights, and fat acceptance. These examples are among the most straightforward in advocating bodily agency, but they also show how the notion of agency can have different meanings. Historians became preoccupied with agency in the 1960s and 1970s, as part of their wish to give labourers a place in social history. A decade later, gender historians especially started from the premise of looking for women's agency in the past.[51] Agency was here defined as the opportunity to shape one's own life, to act independently, even within systems of oppression.

This notion of agency has been criticized, however. Firstly, critics have stated that it is based on a liberal, autonomous subject with choice. Especially with regard to enslaved people or women living under a patriarchal system, it is questionable to what extent they could actually be free subjects in this way. Alternative conceptions of agency include, for instance, interdependence rather than autonomy.[52] A second objection to the liberal notion of agency is that this notion assumes that decisions are based on intentional, rational decision-making, and thus does not accord room to irrational motives or fantasy.[53] Thirdly, it has been pointed out that the notion of the subject with free will is a modern one. Several scholars have therefore called for a historicizing of the notion of agency, in order to make room for other conceptions of agency held in the past.[54] Agency is not necessarily connected to people, for instance. Material qualities can also be ascribed with agency, as occurs in the modern discourse on obesity. Contemporary perceptions of fat people as lacking agency are inextricably connected with older ways of thinking about fat, as Chris Forth argues. Because of fat's encumbering material qualities, it can impede the free movement of the limbs and thus the human will. In antiquity for example, the flabbiness of fat was devalued in contrast to muscular firmness, especially for male bodies. In addition, fat and fattening have been associated in cultural discourse with abject animality, for instance with domesticated animals which are fattened for consumption. Fat itself, Forth maintains, is therefore often attributed agency that forms an obstacle to human intentions.[55]

The focus on rationality and the mind in the classic definition of agency has come at the cost of the body. To include the body in the notion of agency, we can either highlight how people in the past have advocated self-determination of the body, or demonstrate that agency does not revolve only around the mind, but also needs the body. The latter is discussed in Chapter 5 on the experience of the body and embodiment. The present chapter concludes with a discussion of bodily agency as a theme in political movements.

Individual and collective agency with regard to the body has come to the fore primarily in political movements which emphasize body ownership, the right to self-determination, and pride. The most famous example is of course the second feminist wave. 'Body politics' was central to the feminist agenda in the 1960s and 1970s. Feminists debated pornography and discussed whether it was demeaning for women or potentially liberating. They criticized the centrality of men (or **phallocentrism**) in sexuality, advocated the right to abortion, and analyzed rape in relation to patriarchy. One important point made by feminists was that all women should get to know their own bodies better, particularly the functioning of their vaginas. Women were encouraged to take a mirror and simply examine the shape of their vaginas in order to gain more knowledge of their own bodies and their pleasures. The book *Our Bodies Ourselves* (1970, originally titled *Women and their Bodies*), compiled by the Boston Women's Health Collective, presented information on women's health and sexuality, based on empirical evidence as well as women's personal experience with doctors. Covering themes such as abortion, birth control, anatomy, pregnancy, and childbirth, the book was intended to help women gain more knowledge of their own bodies, but also to improve medical healthcare. As the writers explained in their introduction:

> It was exciting to learn new facts about our own bodies, but it was even more exciting to talk about how we felt about our bodies, how we felt about ourselves, how we could become more autonomous human beings, how we could act together on our collective knowledge to change the health care system for women and for all people.[56]

Our Bodies Ourselves was reprinted many times and translated into multiple languages. The translations were adapted to local situations (the Dutch translation of 1975, for instance, added a chapter on lesbian women) and strengthened transnational feminist connections.[57]

In other political movements the self-determination of the body played a major role as well. Civil rights activist and feminist Angela Davis became one of the symbols of the Black Power movement in the 1960s and 1970s, when she proudly wore her big Afro. The 'Black is Beautiful' activists argued for the beauty of the natural black body, refusing to give in to cultural norms regarding white skin or straightened hair.[58] In the disability rights movement, which became especially vocal in the second half of the twentieth century, the rights to autonomy, independence, and self-determination were equally audible. Its aim of attaining legislation which would facilitate the inclusion and empowerment of persons with disabilities, for instance, was already advocated in the 1950s by paralyzed American war veterans. In addition, disability rights activists encouraged people with disabilities to increase their self-esteem and regard their 'disability' as part of a complete self. In this respect, parallels have been drawn with the Black Power movement, and disability has been regarded as beautiful.[59] Particularly, this pride can be found in the deaf community, whose members see themselves as a unique culture that need not be altered or improved. The use of cochlear implants, a technology that allows deaf people to obtain varying degrees of hearing, is opposed by some in the deaf community, who argue that this is a threat to deaf culture.[60]

The body and civil rights were similarly connected in the fat acceptance movement. In 1969 the National Association to Aid Fat Americans (NAAFA) was founded, against the backdrop of the struggle for civil rights. Its aim was to stop discrimination against people perceived as fat and to fight for the acceptance of body fat as a variation of human embodiment. The activists argued against the associations between fat on the one hand and moral weakness and self-inflicted disease on the other. They promoted a view of 'overweight' people as responsible individuals. In the decades that followed, the fat acceptance movement spread from the United States to other countries. It can be argued that these activists evinced two kinds of agency: On the one hand, they fought against discrimination; in this case agency can be seen to lie in resistance against societal norms. On the other hand, activists strove to demonstrate that they were responsible citizens by stating that their body weight did not result from overeating, and by disconnecting fat from disease. In this way, they emphasized that they were healthy, and that in fact it was people who continually dieted and felt unease about their bodies who were the unhealthy ones. As Nora Kreuzenbeck argues, they thus subscribed to a neoliberal ideology of free, responsible, healthy individuals. In addition to resistance, agency could also mean being capable liberal subjects. There were thus two sides to their agency.[61]

To summarize, the feminist, civil, and disability rights movements all centred around bodily agency. Calls for self-acceptance of the natural body went hand in hand with demands for legal bodily self-determination. Protests such as sit-ins or bra burning also involved the active body. Bodily agency could thus imply resistance to the state or the mainstream culture, and the demonstration of a capacity to be a liberal subject deserving of rights.

▶ Conclusion

This chapter has addressed a theoretical perspective that has had a major influence on the history of the body: that of discipline. In the work both of Elias, who writes about the civilizing process, and of Foucault, who speaks of 'docile bodies', the focus lies on new modern disciplining practices with regard to the body. These approaches have many advantages: they show how the treatment of the body is connected to bigger societal processes such as individualization and new forms of power; they also demonstrate how important the body becomes in modern penal practice as well as daily interaction. Scholars have criticized this emphasis on discipline, however, for assuming that the body is passive, a blank slate upon which new societal norms are projected. This presumed lack of agency applies mostly to the early work of Foucault. It has been argued that his emphasis on 'negative subjection' keeps the narrative of the process of subjectification locked in a dialectic of freedom and constraint.[62]

The opposite of discipline seems to be the body politics found in a number of political movements in the second half of the twentieth century – second-wave feminism, the civil and disability rights movement, and the fat acceptance movement – all of which argue for self-determination of the body and protest against the societal disciplining of abnormal bodies.

Several theorists have critiqued the liberal notion of the freely acting subject and have sketched alternative definitions. Similarly, increasingly alternatives are being formulated to the dualist thinking of agency versus discipline. In Chapter 5 we therefore discuss theoretical approaches that concentrate much more on individual bodily experience, which is lacking in theories on discipline and civilization, while Chapter 6 is devoted to recent materialist approaches, which foreground materialist practices with regard to the body, in contrast to the emphasis on powerful discourses often found in theories on discipline. But before we address these new perspectives, we first need to analyze the theories that have impacted the history of the body most strongly: those deriving from social constructionism.

3 The Social Construction of the Body and Disease

▶ Introduction

Bodies have not only been given cultural meaning through, or been shaped by, discipline. In this chapter I focus on social constructionist approaches to the body and disease, of which discipline is only one potential element. As sociologist Chris Shilling defines it: '*social constructionism* is an umbrella term for those views that suggest the body is shaped, constrained, and even invented by society'.[1] The common denominator of social constructionist approaches is that they emphasize that the body (or disease, gender, race, or disability) is culturally constructed. This implies that in different periods and in different places and societies, varying images of the body prevail. In this way, social constructionism argues against biological or **essentialist** approaches, which view the body or sexual differences as fixed and natural. With regard to gender differences, for instance, statements such as 'men's bodies are strong; women's bodies are weak', or 'men are rational; women are emotional' can be considered essentialist since they point to natural, unchanging differences between the sexes. A social constructionist account, on the contrary, would highlight that the differences in bodily strength between men are as variable as the differences in strength between men and women, and that everyone can become stronger with physical training. Similarly, historians have shown how in the eighteenth-century 'cult of sensibility' men were encouraged to cry and were thus seen as emotional creatures. Social constructionists thus highlight cultural and historical changeability.

Often these debates have political meaning: those who argue that there are 'natural' physical differences (between the sexes, for instance, or between races) tend to be conservative, while those who emphasize social constructionism pinpoint social differences in power and historical development, thus also indicating that our views of inequality between people can be changed. Emancipation movements such as the women's liberation movement, the civil rights movement, and the disability rights movement have all been inspired by social constructionist ideas on gender, race, and disability, respectively.

Social constructionism emerged in the latter half of the twentieth century, but the early twentieth century witnessed a number of 'proto social constructionists' – such as cultural Marxists, Weberians, Durkheimian cultural relativists, and symbolical interactionists – who criticized established biological explanations of social inequalities and criminality.[2] Like anthropologists they turned to people's understanding of their lives and their bodies, to classification systems and rituals surrounding the body. A more far-reaching critique of nature and the body as natural entities was put forward by social scientists from the 1960s, and by cultural historians from the 1980s.

The fact that this chapter carries the term 'social construction' in its title does not mean that other chapters in this book do not address theories focusing on the cultural production of the body. In fact, in the previous chapter we have already encountered important social constructionist arguments, such as Foucault's statement that the modern body is disciplined, but also Brigg's emphasis on the social construction of whiteness in her analysis of the discourse on the 'overcivilization' of white women's bodies. The following chapter, moreover, devotes much attention to **postmodern** social constructionist theories in regard to gender and sexuality, formulated for instance by Foucault and Judith Butler. The contribution of this chapter is to explain some of the first theories that together made up the shift towards social constructionism. It starts by outlining anthropological theories that regard the body as a symbolic system and continues with a discussion of social constructionist approaches to disease, which view illnesses as cultural and historical constructions. The chapter concludes by discussing some limitations of social constructionist theories on the body, which are further elaborated in Chapter 6 on materialist approaches to the body.

▶ The body as symbol: Anthropological approaches

Anthropological research has always included discussions of rituals and practices in regard to sexuality and coming of age, in which the body plays a key role. Nevertheless, it was not until the 1970s that the body came to be theorized explicitly in the field of anthropology. **Structuralist** anthropologist Claude Lévi-Strauss (1908–2009) had already noted the importance of tattoos in his study of the Maori, theorizing that tattoos were not simply adornments of the body, but had a deeper meaning: they could be a way to imprint the traditions and beliefs of a group or tribe on the body. For instance, tattoos could indicate the hierarchy of the tribe, clarifying the position of individuals in the group.[3] In this way, Lévi-Strauss pointed to the deeper structures and meanings of certain daily practices that had important functions like communication or establishing relationships.

British anthropologist Mary Douglas (1921–2007) continued Lévi-Strauss's structuralist perspective, but emphasized symbolism (particularly bodily symbolism) even more strongly. Moreover, where Lévi-Strauss took a more universal approach, Douglas preferred to analyze specific cultures. Like Lévi-Strauss, Douglas was interested in systems of classification. In her most famous book, *Purity and Danger* (1966), Douglas interpreted the symbolic meaning of cultural codes in regard to dirt, defilement, and uncleanliness. Arguing against older anthropological work that distinguished 'primitive' from 'civilized' cultures, Douglas emphasized that every culture has its own rules regarding pollution and hygiene. For Douglas, dirt is not a fixed category but should be regarded as 'matter out of place', which gains its meaning by relation to larger symbolic systems of purity and pollution, order and disorder. The distinction between purity and dirt serves to guard borders and preserve moral and cultural order. Often these cultural rules on purity and pollution are applied to the body. Douglas mentions that bodily margins, orifices, and fluids like semen, blood, milk, tears, and excreta are often seen as polluting.[4] In a similar vein, the British anthropologist Edmund Leach (1910–1980) had pointed out that whereas head hair is often carefully groomed, as soon as it is cut off, it is seen as dirt or pollution.[5] Douglas argues that 'the symbolism of the body's boundaries is used [...] to express danger to community boundaries.'[6] In this line of reasoning, emphasizing bodily purity (e.g. the sexual purity of women) or containment is the symbolic equivalent of protecting the purity and coherence of the community.

In the 1980s, cultural historians became interested in working with theories coined by structuralist and symbolic anthropologists. Whereas structuralist anthropologists searched for the ways in which social institutions and relationships served to bolster the social system, symbolic anthropologists, such as Douglas and Clifford Geertz, were more interested in culture as a system of meanings and symbols that needed to be interpreted. However, this distinction between these two kinds of anthropological approaches is somewhat artificial, since they show considerable overlap. Most importantly, cultural historians adopted these anthropologists' focus on the meaning cultural systems gave to all kinds of daily practices, including the care of the body.

One example of the way in which insights from anthropology (in this case symbolic anthropology) can be applied to the history of the body is in regard to menstruation. In the early modern period menstruation was considered a 'barometer of health': in line with humoral thinking, as long as the bodily fluids were in motion, the woman was seen as healthy, but as soon as menstruation halted, this was regarded as a sign of disease. Anthropologists have shown how taboos can apply to menstruating women, who are seen as impure and polluting.[7] In some societies for instance, as Douglas mentions, menstruating women are forbidden to cook.[8] Using this anthropological lens to analyze menstruation in the past, we see that well into the twentieth century, in Europe and America, menstruating women were seen as polluting: It was commonly believed that menstruating women caused meat to go bad, wine to turn, and bread dough to fall.[9]

Another example can be found in early modern thought on masturbation. As historian Michael Stolberg argues, masturbation was regarded as 'waste', since semen was not being used for procreation. Hence, outside the body, spoilt semen was interpreted as 'dirt', in Douglas's definition: matter out of place. It was referred to as the uncleanliness of 'self-pollution'.[10] Similarly, Alison Bashford's study of the Victorian sanitarian discourse shows that it was structured around the dichotomy 'purity vs. pollution'. In their pleas for better hygiene, British doctors often conflated the moral with the physical, as in their description of prostitutes as impure, in contrast to middle-class 'pure' women. Bodies were depicted as houses to be kept clean.[11]

In short, anthropological theories help historians to interpret the symbolism of the body in different cultures, demonstrating that the body only gains meaning in culture and is thus culturally constructed. They also encourage us to look for the deeper meanings of rituals or symbols, pointing to the function of bodily symbolism in certain cultures to establish social order or hierarchy.

▶ The body and illness as metaphor

Similarly to the anthropological focus on the symbolism of the body, several authors have shown how in the West metaphors are used to talk about the body and illness. The American author and cultural critic Susan Sontag (1933–2004), writing in the late 1970s after suffering from cancer, pointed out how our talk of illnesses is always framed by historically changing metaphors, such as the religious connotations of the plague in discussing AIDS or the military metaphor of 'battling cancer'. In medicine, military metaphors first came to be used in the 1880s, when bacteria were identified as agents of disease. Sontag noted that while she had cancer, cancer cells were described as 'invasive' and 'attacking' the body's 'defense', while chemotherapy was equated with chemical warfare.[12] Similarly, in the early twenty-first century, people who die of cancer are frequently said to 'have lost the brave battle', which implies that cancer can be fought as long as the patient is strong enough, and moreover that the individual sufferer has some agency in determining his or her fate. This can be an unfair image, since cancer patients for the most part cannot influence their recovery or response to treatment. Sontag thus underlined that couching illness in metaphorical language could distort the truth about a disease and shame patients. She therefore argued to 'de-mythicize' disease.[13]

The symbolical writing on the body was also pointed out by anthropologist Emily Martin, who scrutinized the metaphors used in scientific accounts of reproductive biology published in English in the 1970s and 1980s. Martin argued that both popular and scientific accounts of the interactions between egg and sperm rely on cultural stereotypes of male and female. Menstruation is often described as a failure, as the death of tissue, whereas the depiction of ovulation uses a vocabulary of passivity, noting that the eggs 'merely sit on the shelf, slowly degenerating and aging like overstocked inventory'.[14] In contrast, sperm are characterized as active, and hence masculinity is associated with productivity and femininity with passivity and destructiveness. Martin points out that scientific language copies cultural stereotypes on gender: the 'feminine' egg is seen as large and passive, the 'masculine' sperm as small, streamlined, and active. Even their meeting is framed as a romance: the egg as 'damsel in distress, shielded only by her sacred garments; sperm as heroic warrior to the rescue'.[15] New research, discovering that the forward thrust of sperm is extremely weak, and the zona (the inner vestments of the egg) functions as an active sperm-catcher, often continued to apply standard gender imagery. Martin aims to excavate the gender stereotypes in scientific writing purportedly presenting the facts of nature, because these biological models can have important social effects.[16] In this sense, metaphors projected onto the body provide us with powerful imagery, with more than 'just language'.

▶ **The social construction of illness: Framing disease**

Not only anthropologists focused on the cultural and metaphorical construction of the body. Sociologists of health and illness, as well as medical historians, became increasingly interested in the social embedding of disease. Whereas the more traditional history of medicine had centred around 'great doctors' and their discoveries, from the 1970s, a social history of medicine was instigated, mostly influenced by protest movements (such as feminism and anti-psychiatry). This social history criticized medicine as paternalistic and anti-democratic and shifted its attention to patients instead of doctors, especially those who were seen to be victims of the medical system such as women, the mad, or the disabled.

In regard to psychiatry, this social history built on critical scholars, who, from the 1950s, attacked institutionalized mental care. Sociologist Erving Goffman (1922–1982) argued in his book *Asylums: Essays on the Social Situation of Mental Patients and other Inmates* (1961) that inmates of asylums were not really mentally ill, but that asylums as 'total institutions' made them so, by taking away their autonomy and forcing them into docile patients. Philosopher Michel Foucault, in his book *Madness and Civilization*, and psychiatrist Thomas Szasz, in his book *The Myth of Mental Illness*, both published in 1961, also criticized modern psychiatric institutions' claim to be humane and to provide cure.[17] Whereas Foucault highlighted how authorities had disciplined – rather than treated – 'mad' patients in the past, Szasz questioned the view of mental illness as a disease, suggesting that 'mental illness was a metaphor, a linguistic strategy that described an offending, disturbing or shocking behaviour'.[18] Rather than an objective scientific category, Szasz argued, mental illness was a social construction and a moral judgement.

These early social constructionist studies of psychiatry influenced the social history of madness, which researched historical change in the treatment of patients suffering from mental illness. Although many historical studies complicated the arguments put forward by Foucault, Foucault's and Szasz's emphasis on the social and professional construction of psychiatric diagnoses would be elaborated by historians of medicine. In the 1980s and 1990s, the history of medicine was influenced by the cultural turn and the central role accorded to especially poststructuralist theory. Now the representation of the body and the ways meaning was made in medicine came to be the central themes.[19]

The American historian of medicine Charles E. Rosenberg, for instance, suggested we research how disease is 'framed', indicating that a disease does not exist as such until it is named. Thus, for Rosenberg the 'act of diagnosis is a key event'.[20] Distinguishing between 'illness' (as a physical condition) and 'disease' (as a social construct), Rosenberg highlighted that disease should be understood in context, as a result of culturally specific behaviour, practices, ideas, and experiences. The most obvious example is the American Psychiatric Association's removal of 'homosexuality' as a pathological condition from the second edition of its *Diagnostic and Statistical Manual* (DSM) in 1973. Rosenberg preferred the term 'framing disease' to 'the social construction of illness', since he found that from the late 1960s to the mid-1980s cultural critics using the term 'social construction' had too often referred to an oppressive social order lying at the heart of social construction.[21] For Rosenberg, the phrase 'framing disease' did not denote this particular critique of power.

An example of the way disease is framed can be taken from the historiography of tuberculosis, now defined as a (potentially deadly) infectious disease caused by bacteria, mostly affecting the lungs and in its active form indicated by symptoms such as a chronic cough with blood-containing sputum, night sweats, fever, and weight loss (the latter symptom forming the basis for its nineteenth-century name 'consumption'). Medical historians have highlighted how the scientist Robert Koch (1843–1910) identified the tuberculosis pathogen in 1882, how the BCG vaccine was first applied to humans in 1921, and how Albert Schatz (1920–2005) found the first effective biomedical treatment in 1944, when he discovered the antibiotic streptomycin. These narratives were primarily based on medical and legislative initiatives to eradicate or contain the disease.[22] Historians working from the perspective of the social and cultural construction of disease, in contrast, sketch the social circumstances of patients, but also tuberculosis' cultural associations and its changing definition. Historical research has shown how in the early twentieth century the image of the 'careless consumptive' surfaced, which was associated with immigrants, alcoholics, and homeless people who did not take sufficient care of themselves and had to be cured with incarceration, isolation, and hygiene.[23] Not only were consumption sufferers, especially lower-class patients, often regarded as 'dirty', they were also stigmatized by families and communities.[24]

Apart from describing the social circumstances of tuberculosis patients, historians have also pointed to the stereotypes of those sufferers. In nineteenth-century literature and painting, consumption was represented as the 'romantic disease': it was seen to help artistic talent, probably since consumption's slight fever and the presence of toxins in the blood was considered to provide the sufferer with wise insights into human existence. Whereas in nineteenth-century literature the stereotype of the gentle, white, female invalid was paramount, and disease and death rates therefore tended to exclude non-white people, in contemporary society the immigrant sweatshop worker is the stereotypical tuberculosis patient. And while nineteenth-century artists and authors located consumption in 'evocative settings such as the orphanage, madhouse, poorhouse, inner sanctum, riverboat, and woodlot',[25] these locations are no longer associated with tuberculosis. Historian Katherine Ott therefore concludes: 'What we call "tuberculosis" was not the same disease in 1850 that it was in 1900 or even 1950'.[26] The history of this disease chronicles the shift from a romantic, indistinct illness to a clearly and biomedically defined disease, treated with high-tech and strongly connected with public health and hygiene. For Ott, consumption and tuberculosis were different diseases.[27]

Social constructionist approaches to the history of illness thus emphasize the cultural and historical variation of disease and the body. These approaches have, however, led to scholarly debate on the exact nature of the relationship between the biological essence of a disease and its cultural construction. We will further explore this debate by looking at the examples of hysteria and anorexia nervosa.

▶ The history of hysteria

Hysteria has received ample attention from both medical and cultural historians for several reasons. Firstly, its prevalence among the middle and upper classes in the nineteenth century was very conspicuous, not least from famous novels such as Gustave Flaubert's *Madame Bovary* (published in 1856). Secondly, hysteria's increasing popularity in the eighteenth and especially the nineteenth century contrasted sharply with its sudden disappearance around the First World War. This suggested the conclusion that hysteria was merely a fashionable occurrence, not a real disease. To begin, we therefore need to answer two questions: What is hysteria? And how should historians interpret this phenomenon?

Hysteria can refer to many different symptoms, such as emotional fits, irritability, headaches, fainting, bodily insensitivity, and paralysis. From antiquity on, doctors and later psychiatrists debated the causes of this disease, mostly discussing whether its origin was located in the body or the mind, as well as whether men too could suffer from hysteria. In antiquity women's hysteria was connected with the uterus, the 'wandering womb' that could cause problems in other body parts. In the course of the seventeenth century, the locus of hysteria shifted from the reproductive system to the nerves and the brain. The idea of male hysteria now became a possibility.[28] The late eighteenth and early nineteenth centuries saw a revival of gynaecological theories of hysteria, which became dominant. Especially in the second half of the nineteenth century, physicians vehemently debated the origin and location of hysteria. One of the foremost doctors who carried out research into hysteria was the French neurologist Jean-Martin Charcot (1825–1893). Charcot relied on degeneration theories, stating that from birth hysterics had a latent defect of the nervous system, which was later triggered by a traumatic incident of some kind (such as physical illness, alcoholism, or workplace accidents), hence also the term 'traumatic hysteria'. Charcot's case histories began with the search for hereditary antecedents, even though the exact relationship between hysteria and degeneration was debated by many physicians. Charcot was a materialist and continued to look for the organic cause of hysteria, although he never found it. His work, based on case studies, was descriptive and mostly aimed at classification.[29]

For Charcot the most conspicuous hallmarks of hysteria were the aberrations of sensibility: the hysterical stigmata, like anaesthesias (lack of sensitivity) and hyperaesthesias (exaggerations of sensibility), and abnormalities of the five senses (mostly visual disturbances). A second major category of symptoms were the motor impairments. Furthermore, for Charcot hysteria was connected with respiratory, digestive, and language disorders. The 'hysterogenic zones' were a hallmark of French hysteria theory: these were pressure points that could lead to a hysterical aura and then a hysterical fit. They could be found anywhere on the body, including in the groin or genitalia (in both men and women).

Charcot's model of hysteria was accepted by the mainstream medical world in Europe in the 1870s and 1880s. From 1878 to 1893 Charcot also examined male hysteria. The men Charcot labelled with hysteria were mostly working men. As the historian Mark Micale argues, for Charcot, in principle hysteria was the same for men and women. The French doctor found gender differences only in a few respects, notably the frequency (the male to female ratio was 1:20), and the idea that women were the sole parental agents of direct transmission of hysteria to their sons. This meant that hysteria remained a disease primarily associated with women. Most importantly, the secondary causes were thought to differ by gender: women were most commonly triggered into hysteria by strong emotions such as marital turmoil, unrequited love, religious ecstasy, superstitious fear, or death of a relative. These mostly refer to domestic settings. By contrast, the male hysterics often developed hysteria after a physically traumatic incident (for instance a workplace accident), and it was compounded by prior venereal infection or alcoholic excess. When it came to emotions, hysteria in the male was mainly associated with 'manly' emotions such as rage, jealousy, and agitation. Women thus fell ill due to their vulnerable emotional natures and inability to control their feelings, while men's suffering was triggered by working, drinking, and fornicating too much. Charcot also described the symptoms in gender-specific terms, as Micale shows. While for the male patients Charcot used mainly somatic terms, with little attention for mental elements, for female patients he prioritized emotional states. Generally, however, there were more similarities than differences between the genders.[30]

After Charcot, many other doctors and psychiatrists would debate the origins of hysteria, most of them, for example Freud, emphasizing its mental genesis, which then caused the physical symptoms. Most historians argue that after the First World War hysteria slowly disappeared. Micale notes two common explanations: firstly, the idea that it was de-Victorianization (the disappearance of repression) that caused hysteria to vanish. However, the chronology does not fit: sexual liberation took place for a large part after the war, by which time hysteria is already supposed to have disappeared. A second explanation suggests that once patients began to understand the psychology behind hysteria, it no longer worked as a strategy. This explanation assumes that before the twentieth century, people easily and unconsciously converted emotional distress into somatic symptoms, whereas with the coming of the 'psychological society' and its broadly shared knowledge of the workings of psychosomatic illness, this **somatization** of anxieties decreased in effectiveness since it was recognized by both professionals and laypeople. There is, however, little evidence to back this up. Micale proposes another explanation: taking a medical-historical perspective, he argues that the diagnosis of hysteria underwent such major reformulations between 1895 and 1910 that hysteria as such was no longer recognizable as a concept. Hysteria shifted from a unitary disease category to a secondary psychological reaction that could accompany any physical or mental disorder. Moreover, the former hysteria diagnosis was absorbed by new categories coined by modern psychosomatic medicine, which emerged in the second quarter of the twentieth century, such as epilepsy, psychosis, and neurosis.[31]

Similarly, contemporary neurologists argue that it is not so much the symptoms of hysteria (such as paralysis or blackouts) that disappeared as the twentieth century progressed, but medical interest in the condition: hysteria was neglected by both psychiatrists and neurologists. Some of its symptoms now live on under new diagnostic categories such as 'conversion disorder', which refers to neurological symptoms, for example paralysis, which cannot be explained by organic causes, but are triggered by psychologically stressful situations.[32]

These interpretations stress that hysteria has some basic material symptoms, caused or triggered by mental problems, which have been labelled differently in different periods. This would imply that hysteria is not a complete cultural construct, simply given different names over time. Other historians tend to emphasize the cultural influence more, and regard hysteria primarily as a cultural phenomenon rather than a disease. Some feminist scholarship, for instance, views hysteria as a feminist protest against Victorian patriarchal restrictions. These scholars highlight the secondary gains of being ill. The American historian Carroll Smith-Rosenberg, for instance, regards hysteria as a social role within the nineteenth-century family, a passive form of resistance against patriarchy's limitation of women's possibilities:

> The discontinuity between the roles of courted woman and pain-bearing, self-sacrificing wife and mother, the realities of an unhappy marriage, the loneliness and chagrin of spinsterhood may all have made the petulant infantilism and narcissistic self-assertion of the hysteric a necessary alternative to women who felt unfairly deprived of their promised social role and who had few strengths with which to adapt to a more trying one.

Smith-Rosenberg concludes that the hysterical woman 'can be seen as both product and indictment of her culture'.[33]

To summarize, historical explanations of hysteria vary from interpreting it as a disease, with a mental origin and somatic symptoms, that was given different names over time, to a purely cultural construction, which disappeared when the social circumstances changed.

▷ The history of anorexia nervosa

We can ask the same questions with regard to the diagnosis of anorexia nervosa, nowadays regarded as a disease or disorder, although its causes and cures are strongly contested. A historical perspective might help us understand anorexia better. Women who starve themselves have been known since the Middle Ages. One famous example is Saint Catherine of Siena (1347–1380), who was attributed with miraculous visions in which she experienced a mystical marriage with Christ. She died of starvation at the age of 33. In the Middle Ages, refusing food or being unable to eat took place in a religious context, in which denial of the body implied a spiritual connection with God. Fasting was 'fundamental to the model of female holiness'.[34] In later centuries, this miraculously inspired loss of appetite would be termed 'anorexia mirabilis'.

Modern anorexia is less shaped by religion. The diagnosis 'anorexia nervosa' was coined in 1873 by the British doctor William Withey Gull, while in the same year the French neurologist Charles Lasègue came up with the term 'anorexie hystérique'. Anorexia now gained its own label and became medicalized and part of the group of 'nervous diseases'. Gull associated it with adolescent girls and with hysteria. For him, these young women were suffering from a morbid mental state leading to emaciation. Lasègue emphasized the family environment conducive to anorexia. In nineteenth-century France, as in other European countries, middle-class sons and daughters increasingly lived with their parents until they married. They were more dependent on their families than children from the working classes. This period of adolescence led to an intensification of family life and parental scrutiny. Lasègue noticed that adolescent girls from the bourgeoisie had the power to disrupt their families by refusing to eat, food symbolizing parental love par excellence. The French physician attributed the cause of this behaviour to emotion and frustration connected with the transition to adulthood, such as struggles with parents or inappropriate romantic hopes.[35]

Historian Joan Jacobs Brumberg criticizes those medical writers and historians who see the medieval anorexia mirabilis and modern anorexia nervosa as manifestations of the same disease. This biological explanation is too simplistic, Brumberg argues, and does not take into account the vastly different cultural circumstances. However, Brumberg does not resort solely to cultural constructionism; instead she proposes an explanatory model that combines biological, psychological, and cultural explanations. She points out that biomedical experiences also play a role, for instance as the anorectic patient slowly becomes addicted to starvation and becomes physically unable to eat. Furthermore, psychological models that focus on patterns of interaction in families, and on anorexia as a pathological response to problems of adolescence, are helpful yet not sufficient. Arguing for the reciprocity of biology and culture, Brumberg finds approaches that regard anorexia as a 'mere social construction' deficient: she is critical of feminist authors who, rather than seeing anorexia as a disease, regard it as a conscious political protest against patriarchy. For Brumberg, this approach ignores the fact that anorectics suffer from a dangerous disease. Moreover, it does not explain why not all women resort to this type of protest.[36]

Brumberg's combination of biological, psychological, and cultural models has not convinced everyone, however. For instance, feminist philosopher Susan Bordo rejects the opposition between interpreting anorexia as either a disease or a political protest, since this opposition loses sight of the political meaning of a cultural analysis. Bordo's own cultural analysis focuses on finding meaning in the demands culture has placed on women. Similarly to the self-mortification of the medieval women who starved themselves, modern anorexia, Bordo claims, has a deeply spiritual dimension: 'in the context of enduring historical traditions that have dominantly coded appetite, lack of will, temptation, and, indeed, the body itself as female, surely we would expect that women's projects to transcend hunger and desire would reveal some continuous elements'.[37] Bordo does not aim primarily at reconstructing historical continuums, but prioritizes a cultural, political analysis over a medical one that would present doctors as the only experts.

Similarly to the history of hysteria, then, historical explanations of anorexia vary from regarding it as a purely cultural construction to classifying it as a disease, although there seems to be more historical continuity in the occurrence of anorexia than of hysteria. Brumberg's design of an explanatory model that includes biological, psychological, and cultural elements aims to take historical research beyond an 'either disease or cultural construction' interpretation.

▶ The history of disability

The social construction of the body comes to the fore with particular prominence in the field of disability studies. Already in 1963 sociologist Erving Goffman wrote a book on stigma: the experiences of people considered by society as abnormal, such as physically deformed people, mental patients, prostitutes, or drug addicts. However, it was only in the 1980s that disability studies were founded as a new discipline, strongly influenced by gender studies in its focus on ability as an identity category. While gender scholars highlighted the dichotomy sex-gender, disability studies centred on the dichotomy impairment-disability. Disability scholars distinguish between a 'medical' and a 'social' model of disability, the medical referring to a physical impairment, such as having only one leg or having been born with Down syndrome. In this medical model physicians regard the disabled individual as not conforming to the norm of 'health' and try to 'repair' the body by, for instance, constructing artificial limbs or hearing devices. The social model of disability, by contrast, argues against any biological or fixed impairment and instead stresses that whom society terms 'disabled' is culturally constructed and historically variable. A person in a wheelchair may be seen as disabled, whereas this person considers himself or herself perfectly able to do many things. The social model of disability emphasizes that disability is first and foremost a social problem, defined by medical doctors or society and effectively disqualifying numerous people. An analysis of disability thus leads to a critical view of the distinction between 'normal' and 'deformed' or 'disabled' bodies and to a plea for human diversity.[38]

Historians have shown how the definition of disability has changed over time. Until the twentieth century, people with physical deformities, such as bearded women or 'dwarfs', were often displayed in freak shows and labelled as monsters. They were viewed with both horror and awe, as they were also regarded as miracles of nature or evidence of divine power. From the nineteenth century on, a medicalized notion of disability emerged, defining disability as a personal physical deficit in need of medical correction. The strong emphasis on the norm and average stems only from the mid-nineteenth century.[39] The twentieth century witnessed a strong exclusion (sometimes even annihilation) of people who did not meet the eugenicist standard of fitness, as reflected for instance in the forced sterilization of deaf or intellectually disabled individuals. At the same time, that century saw the establishment of many organizations that advocated disabled people's rights, such as the League of the Physically Handicapped, which was founded in the United States in 1935.[40] Yet the disability rights movement only really gained momentum from the 1960s and came to impact legislation especially in the 1980s.

In their social constructionist analyses, disability scholars demonstrate how disability intersects with other identity categories. As Rosemarie Garland-Thomson writes: 'the representational systems of gender, race, ethnicity, ability, sexuality and class mutually construct, inflect, and contradict one another'.[41] Garland-Thomson shows how black people were often labelled as disabled. For example, the Khoikhoi woman Sarah Baartman was taken from South Africa, enslaved, sold, and put on display as the 'Hottentot Venus' in London and Paris in 1810. Her body, especially her breasts, buttocks, and hypertrophied labia, aroused considerable interest from both the general public and from scientists. She was exhibited as a freak, much like the other 'living curiosities' on display in London shows, such as 'dwarfs', living skeletons, and obese people. She was treated as an object, and no documents in her own voice have survived.[42] As Rosemarie Garland-Thomson argues, this racial and gender degradation was framed in a language of abled/disabled, Baartman's racial and gender corporeal hallmarks being presented to a white European audience as deformities.[43] The intersection of ethnicity and disability also surfaced in the discourses surrounding American immigration in the first decades of the twentieth century, when proponents of the restriction of immigration were convinced of the physical inferiority of southern-European and Jewish immigrants. Immigration officials picked out people with visible 'abnormalities'. This measure was meant to determine who was able to work, but had strong eugenicist connotations, stressing the wish for a 'pure' American people.[44]

The comparison between disability as a marker of identity with identity categories such as gender, ethnicity, class, and sexuality raises the question whether all these categories function in the same way. Some critics have stated that the material body plays a more important and inescapable element in regard to disability than in the forming of gender or racial identities. Isn't pain, for example, an indicator of the physical limits to social construction? Some disabled groups even strive after official disability recognition, such as patients suffering from chronic fatigue syndrome (CFS/ME). Here, the social stigma is appropriated by disabled people and used to their own advantage. Another question raised is whether the diverse experiences of being disabled can be grouped under one heading. Not only is it difficult to compare physical impairments with mental diseases, also the analysis of the 'ability/disability system' might not be the same as an analysis of individual experiences.[45]

▸ Conclusion

In this overview of social constructionist theories of the body, disease, and disability, we have seen that there are different 'gradations' of social constructionism. On the one hand there are scholars who regard the body or disease as completely constructed by culture. This applies for example to most proponents of the social model of disability and to some feminist explanations of hysteria and anorexia. On the other hand we can group those historians, anthropologists, and other scholars who, though they would not claim that the body or disease has no biological component at all, are simply interested in how diseases are labelled and how these frames change over time. This is the stance, for instance, of the medical historian Charles Rosenberg. Several historians, such as Joan Jacobs Brumberg in her study on anorexia, advocate an explanatory model that includes the intricate ways in which biology, psychology, and culture interact.

The preference for culture or biology as an explanatory model is connected to the aim of the researcher or activist. Philosopher Ian Hacking has pointed out the differences in the agendas of social constructionists. Whereas all social constructionists start from the premise that X (race, gender, disability) is not inevitable, not determined by the nature of things, some of them go one step further and state that X is bad and should be abolished or radically transformed.[46] Moreover, the political ideas of essentialists and social constructionists do not always follow directly from their views: although **essentialism** is very often a crutch for sexism or racism, this need not be the case.[47]

Apart from the realization that there are different gradations and agendas within social constructionism, several criticisms have been advanced. Firstly, as Hacking points out, social constructionist theories often lack clarity about what exactly is constructed, and by whom. Referring to books and discussions on the social construction of race, gender, madness, the economy, modern science, the self, and the environment, to name but a few, which he feels have become omnipresent in both the academic fields of history and social science and in political discourse, Hacking argues that they sometimes confuse a concept with the objects that fall under it. For example, western government institutions classify 'women refugees' as such, thus making them into a bureaucratic category. This classification can have a real impact on women refugees' lives, but it is the concept 'refugee women', rather than the women themselves, that is socially constructed here.[48] In addition to a clear definition of what exactly is being constructed, some of these social constructionist theories are not clear about who or what is doing the constructing. As we saw above, the medical historian Charles Rosenberg thought the concept of social construction reeked too much of a controlling, oppressive social order and hence preferred the term 'framing' (disease). In general terms, social construction can refer to a tyrannical and unjust society as agent, but also simply to a social system that generates meaning. Some social constructionist theorists (poststructuralists, as we shall see in the next chapter) regard linguistic categories as *determinant* of our bodily experiences, while others state that people have the agency to give meaning to their bodies with the help of cultural symbols.

Secondly, and connected to the first objection, we might ask whether the body or disease is socially constructed 'top down', or throughout society or even 'bottom up'. Many theories remain vague about how pervasive this process of construction actually is. This is why Hacking has introduced the concept of the 'looping effect of human kinds' to indicate that a label (e.g. 'disabled') is not only imposed top down (as social constructionism often assumes), but also has to be taken up or rejected by individuals, who, moreover, change it while using it and thus provide feedback that can alter the label (hence 'looping effects').[49] Medical historians too have advocated combining top-down and bottom-up approaches, as in the interaction between physicians and patients.[50]

Thirdly, it has been objected that social constructionism in general is too relativist and leaves too little space for any foundations. If knowledge of the body and disease are historically changeable, what foundational insights *can* we rely on, and is progress possible at all? This objection often relies on a caricatured image of social constructionism, whose critics impute to it the claim that diseases are not real and that science and medicine are ineffective.[51] In fact, social constructionism does not deny that there are standards, but aims to show that they are historically variable.[52]

A fourth and related criticism concerns the material aspects of the body: Do cultural constructionists not lose sight of the material body and the biological essence of disease? It is certainly true that social constructionism highlights the cultural framing and historical change of body images, but this does not necessarily imply that the material aspects of the body are denied. Rather, as historian Ludmilla Jordanova states: 'the material world is constantly shaped and interpreted through human actions and consciousness'.[53] However, other methodologies seem to be better suited to demonstrating these material sides of the body, as we will see in Chapter 6.

To conclude with a few insights that social constructionism has provided, we might point to its focus on historical and cultural change, especially in regard to topics that previously seemed unchanging (sexual or racial differences, for instance). Jordanova suggests that the great contribution of social constructionism to the history of medicine 'has been to make historians think much harder about processes and interactions that were previously invisible, denied, or thought unproblematic.'[54] The critical nature of social constructionist theories of the body and disease have made us aware of the impact of changing ideologies on the sexed, raced, and disabled body.[55]

4 The Body, Gender, and Sexuality

▶ Introduction

This chapter builds on the previous chapter in discussing how social constructionist theories can be applied to the study of gender, sexuality, and the body.
The work of historians in this field will be compared with feminist, gender, and
queer theory. This chapter focuses on two main themes: firstly, the question of
whether sexual difference (or the idea that two kinds of bodies exist, that is, male
and female) is culturally constructed, and if so, how views have changed over
time; and secondly, the issue of how we can theorize the relationships between
sex, gender, and desire, and how these relationships may have varied in the
course of history.

The first section of this chapter introduces the work of the historian Thomas
Laqueur, who traces the development from the early-modern one-sex system to
the modern two-sex system in order to demonstrate that bodily sex is a cultural
construct. The second section concentrates on the various body parts – varying
from genitals, gonads, hormones, and chromosomes, to the brain – that historians have, at different moments of history, regarded as the unequivocal seat of
femininity or masculinity. The chapter then shifts the focus to the theme of the
body in feminist, gender, and queer theory, including the work of Simone de
Beauvoir, Michel Foucault, and Judith Butler. These theorists all problematize
the relationships between the body, gender, and sexuality. At the end of the
chapter queer history is compared with queer theory, to show that a historical
approach to gender and sexuality often reaches similar conclusions to those of
gender and queer theory.

▶ Laqueur and the shift to the two-sex system

In the 1980s, gender historians such as Joan Scott proposed that rather than looking at the lives of women in the past, historians should apply the notion of 'gender', the social and cultural construction of masculinity and femininity.[1] This focus on the cultural discourses of femininity and masculinity implied that the body was a blank slate, upon which cultural ideology was projected. As anthropologist Gayle Rubin had already noted in 1975: 'Every society also has a sex/gender system – a set of arrangements by which the biological raw material of human sex and procreation is shaped by human, social intervention and satisfied in a conventional manner.'[2] Like Rubin, many early gender historians grouped the body under 'biological raw material', which was seen as less interesting to study than the social arrangements that formulated gender norms and practices.

This lack of attention to the body in gender history changed with the influential book by the American historian Thomas Laqueur (1945–), *Making Sex: Body and Gender from the Greeks to Freud* (1990), which showed that not only gender, but also the body, was socially constructed. Laqueur argued that humoralism involved a 'one-sexed body': rather than there being two separate sexes, doctors from antiquity to the early modern period believed that only one sex existed, and that the female anatomy was simply an underdeveloped, less perfect version of the fully realized male body. The humoralist doctrine taught that male bodies were hot and dry, and that female bodies were cold and moist. This difference in temperature and constitution stimulated the growth of male genitals on the outside of the body, whereas the female genitals remained on the inside. Remarkably, in this view all genitals had the same shape: the vagina (or 'the neck of the womb') was regarded as an inverted penis, and the uterus was seen as corresponding to the scrotum; both men and women were thought to have testes (what we now call ovaries were referred to as 'female testicles'). Similarly, in the early modern humoral system menstruation in females was seen as analogous to a male nose bleed: since both sexes were regarded as having corresponding corporeal flows, menstruation did not yet function as designator of the female body.[3]

Laqueur argues that it was only at the end of the eighteenth century that his one-sex system came to be replaced by a two-sex system that closely resembled our present-day assumptions about the existence of two opposite sexes, male and female. Laqueur only partially attributed this change to the new scientific discoveries of that era, which revealed the differences between male and female genitals. Instead, he showed that these medical discoveries – emerging knowledge of the anatomy of the male and female body, the cycle of ovulation, the production of sperm, conception, menstruation, and, later, in the 1920s and 1930s, the role of hormones in reproduction – were not enough to make people see two fundamentally different bodies. This shift was primarily caused by cultural and political change, including the Enlightenment, which promoted equality between all people, including between men and women. In response to this imminent – and threatening – equality between the sexes, Laqueur states, doctors started to emphasize anatomical differences based on sex: the 'discovery' that the female brain was smaller was used as evidence of women's incapacity to function in the public sphere, and their broader hips were a hallmark sign of women's destiny to give birth.[4]

From the late eighteenth century, anatomists drew detailed illustrations of the female skeleton for the first time; previously there had only been one basic structure. By depicting a skeletal ostrich with a huge pelvis in the background of his drawing of the female skeleton, and a horse behind the male skeleton, the Scottish anatomist John Barclay (1758–1826) directed the viewer's attention to the human female's pelvis. As historian Londa Schiebinger notes, these drawings, published posthumously in 1829, contrasted the symbolic masculinity of the horse, denoting speed, power, and endurance, with a 'natural' motherhood figured by the ostrich's wide hips. In another drawing Barclay inserted a child's skeleton in between the male and the female, to accentuate the similarities between the child's skull size, bones, rib cage, jaw shape, and feet size and those of the female skeleton.[5] In short, women's bodies were associated with motherhood and compared to children, thus emphasizing the inequality between men and women.

By the mid-nineteenth century, male and female were seen as two completely different sexes. Laqueur's central argument is that bodily sex is culturally variable; we might think that because of a lack of scientific discoveries, the one-sex system simply did not see the body in the same way current science has shown it to be. But Laqueur states that 'seeing is believing': in any era, we observe with culturally tinted spectacles. The one-sex system was not biologically grounded, but part of cultural ideas on gender that determined how people saw the body. Laqueur's important contribution to the history of the body was to point out that the body itself has a history and that, instead of taking a biologically sexed body as a starting point, we should first consider looking at cultural ideas on gender (masculinity–femininity), since they also determine how we view the body.

Laqueur's book has not been without criticism, however. Firstly, several historians have argued against the universal presence of the one-sex model in antiquity and the Middle Ages, citing the conflict among ancient and medieval authorities in regard to gender difference, on the one hand, and demonstrating the presence of the two-sex model long before the Enlightenment, on the other.[6] Michael Stolberg for instance presents medical writings dating from around 1600 which prove that leading physicians had already noted sexual differences in anatomy.[7] Secondly, Laqueur's choice to focus primarily on anatomical texts has been criticized, since it tells us little about how the body was understood by ordinary people.[8] Thirdly, other historians have shown that in medical *practice*, bodily differences played a major role in the treatment of male and female patients already in the seventeenth and eighteenth centuries.[9] This historical writing thus attests an awareness of sexual differences in the period in which, according to Laqueur, the one-sex system reigned supreme. Lastly, it has been questioned whether the male body was really the cultural paradigm, the norm against which the mysterious, unruly female body was measured. Cathy McClive censures 'the imposition of a single, dominant interpretation of masculinity, and indeed of the male body, at the expense of a more nuanced picture of embodied masculinities'.[10] McClive states, on the basis of seventeenth- and eighteenth-century French court records, in which the bodies of hermaphrodites were examined, that the functioning of the penis was tested and the excretions from the body were scrutinized. McClive therefore argues that

> Gender did not override sex, as Laqueur has argued, but an individual's corporeal reality was what determined his or her place in society. Male genitalia did not always make the man in early modern France, but a functioning penis capable of erection, penetration and the ejaculation of fertile seed could.[11]

In contrast to Laqueur's argument that gender overrode sex in the early modern period, patriarchal norms on masculinity such as control of the family were, according to McClive, directly linked to the male body via proof of physical potency through the engendering of progeny in marriage.

To summarize, these historians suggest that sexual differences played a bigger role in early modern society than Laqueur claimed, and that the male body was not regarded as perfect as in medical theory. Moreover, questions have been raised about Laqueur's positioning of gender as primary, determining sex.

▷ **The location of sexual difference in history**

Whereas Laqueur and Schiebinger focused mainly on the genitals and the skeleton, other scholars have researched different indicators of sexual disparity in history, which primarily relate to reproduction. In the nineteenth century especially, women were seen as governed by their wombs. From the 1840s the ovaries specifically were seen to be the ultimate cause of women's otherness.[12] Since they were thought to be dominated by their reproductive function, women were qualified as more physical, instinctual, and emotional than men, and 'womanhood' was equated with 'pathology'.[13] As part of the model of the human body as a closed system containing a fixed quantity of energy, women were represented as continuously internally unstable. Their 'innate periodicity' was seen to directly correspond to mental disorders like hysteria.[14]

Menstruation played a pivotal role in contemporary debates on the hallmarks of femininity. During the eighteenth century, medical belief in the existence of male menstruation was already declining.[15] It was, however, only in the nineteenth century – with the arrival of a **solidist** model of the body, which focused on the organs and their specific functions as explanations for menstruation, rather than on the moving fluids at the centre of the holistic humoralist view – that menstruation grew to be the 'outstanding token of femininity and sexual difference'.[16] Whereas in early modern medical theory menstruation had been seen as a sign of health since it evacuated superfluous blood, in the middle of the nineteenth century it became an indicator of fertility. A new model equated menstruation to ovulation (the fertile period coinciding with the peak of sexual desire), thereby putting humans and animals on the same footing, since they were both considered to be 'on heat'.[17] At the end of the nineteenth century, medical discourse started to emphasize yet another aspect of menstruation; it was thought to parallel disease. The fact that women menstruated now implied they were ill once a month and prone to debility in general, and therefore also unfit for public office and higher education.[18]

It was not until about 1930 that western doctors came to regard menstruation as a sign of non-pregnancy, since the relationship between menstruation and ovulation had now been clarified. In the 1920s and 1930s the emerging field of endocrinology had discovered the workings of hormones. These scientific findings lie at the basis of the modern hormonal body. Initially, endocrinologists thought there was only one hormone per sex, but later they observed that both sexes produced 'male' (testosterone) and 'female' (oestrogen) hormones. This chemical model of sex and the body implied that sex was an entity that could exist apart from any fixed location in the body. Femininity was no longer located in the uterus or ovaries, masculinity no longer in the testes; rather sex was thought to develop in a complex feedback system between the gonads and the brain. Nelly Oudshoorn has referred to this new model of the hormonal body as potentially revolutionizing the ideas on biological sex:

> The model suggested that, chemically speaking, all organisms are both male and female [...] In this model, an anatomical male could possess feminine character-istics controlled by female sex hormones, while an anatomical female could have masculine characteristics regulated by male sex hormones.[19]

Nevertheless, this revolutionary potential seems not to have been fulfilled. For all its innovation, including the introduction of technical tools such as hormo-nal blood tests, the hormonal model did not fully replace the dualistic two-sex model. Firstly, this sexual dichotomy was preserved by the conceptualization of sex differences in terms of the rhythm of hormone production. Gynaecologists characterized the female body by its cyclic hormonal regulation, and the male body by its stable hormonal regulation. This focus on cyclicity moreover built on older notions of the female body: already in the second half of the nine-teenth century, psychiatrists had associated femininity with cyclicity by linking the 'periodic madness' of their female patients to menstruation. The hormone model also accentuated the image of the female body as primarily a reproduc-tive body.[20] Thus, the discovery of sex hormones provided new ways of classify-ing male and female bodies, but at the same time was also influenced by older notions of dualistic sex differences.

A similar argument can be found in the study of chromosomes, another potential indicator of bodily sex. In her study of the medical treatment of 'inter-sex' children (children born with ambiguous sexual characteristics, previously termed 'hermaphrodites'), Anne Fausto-Sterling highlights the medical 'need' to immediately assign one of only two sexes to the baby, a practice that has been especially common since the 1950s. She also asks why, given that there are more than two possible pairs of sex chromosomes (not just XX and XY, for instance, but also XO and XXY), doctors and society do not allow for more than just two categories when it comes to bodily sex.[21] Fausto-Sterling therefore concludes that 'labeling someone a man or a woman is a social decision'.[22]

In short, in the nineteenth century especially doctors searched for the 'seat of femininity', mostly locating this seat in the womb or the ovaries, in menstruation, and from around 1930 in sex hormones. This historical overview demonstrates that the sexed body is culturally and historically variable: what counts as a female body differs. Whereas gender historians in the 1980s neglected the body, historian Laqueur placed it centre stage. However, Laqueur too pointed primarily to ideas on gender to explain how the body was perceived. To further explore these complex interconnections between gender and the body, I will now turn to feminist, gender, and queer theory.

▶ The body in feminist theory: Simone de Beauvoir's *The Second Sex*

Early feminists already discussed the female body. Mary Wollstonecraft (1759–1797), for example, complained that society forced women to be too preoccupied with beauty and fashion, thus making a 'gilt cage' of their bodies.[23] However, it was only in the twentieth century, especially during the second feminist wave in the 1970s, that the body began to attract central attention in feminist theory. An influential precursor to the second feminist wave was Simone de Beauvoir's existentialist analysis of women's lives, *The Second Sex*, published in 1949.

De Beauvoir argued that western culture regarded only men as full persons, conscious of the possibilities of self-creation and able to make decisions, whereas women were mostly regarded as the Other, without options for self-transformation, the ultimate goal of the philosophy of **existentialism**. The famous French philosopher thought women should transcend their links to nature in order to overcome this status as the Other. In her view, the position of women as 'the second sex' derived partly from their reproductive capacity and (socially prescribed) task of taking care of children. It was society that was responsible for allocating women this part to play: 'One is not born, but rather becomes, woman'.[24] The female body was from de Beauvoir's perspective alienating: 'woman *is* her body as man *is* his but her body is something other than her'.[25] Pregnancy denied women the chance to steer their own lives freely:

> Ensnared by nature, the pregnant woman is plant and animal, a stock-pile of colloids, an incubator, an egg; she scares children proud of their young, straight bodies and makes young people titter contemptuously because she is a human being, a conscious and free individual, who has become life's passing instrument.[26]

De Beauvoir considered every biological process in the female body – such as menstruation, childbirth, and menopause – a 'crisis' or a 'trial', resulting in **alienation**. Women's bodies prevented them from asserting their own subjectivity. In her view, the authentic male body, especially male erotic desire, led to full subjectivity, whereas the female body was sexually passive: 'Feminine heat is the flaccid palpitation of a shellfish; where man has impetuousness, woman merely has impatience [...] she, like a carnivorous plant, waits for and watches the swamp where insects and children bog down.'[27]

De Beauvoir's book is an indictment against patriarchy, which kept women in a subordinate position, yet her negative depictions of the female body sometimes border on essentialist disgust. As Toril Moi argues, de Beauvoir's account of female sexuality is phallocentric, taking male sexuality as the ideal and distinguishing between a male active body and female, passive 'flesh'. However, the historical background at the time of her writing – the lack of contraception and prohibition of abortion in France in the 1940s – might also explain the French philosopher's negative view of female sexuality.[28] In short, *The Second Sex* paradoxically combines an essentialist view of the debilitating female body and a social constructionist perspective of woman as the Other. It is the latter argument that has influenced later feminist theory.

The originally Marxist concept of alienation that de Beauvoir worked with later resurfaced in much socialist feminist writing of the 1970s, which emphasized women's alienation from their bodies: just as male wageworkers regarded their bodies as mere machines from which labour power was extracted, women's bodies, from a socialist feminist perspective, were objects that were worked on, for example by plucking eyebrows. And just as wageworkers were in competition with each other, women competed with other women for male approval.[29]

In conclusion, most feminist theory since de Beauvoir has started from the premise that femininity is a cultural construction. Her book has been read by many women as an opportunity of envisioning a different future for women and their bodies.[30] De Beauvoir's negative and essentialist view of the female body and female sexuality, however, did not find its way into later feminist theory.

▶ Foucault and the history of sexuality

At the time of the second feminist wave and the gay liberation movement, sexuality was prominent on the agenda. Both historians and other theorists started to address the history of sexuality. A key influence in this field was Foucault's publication of the first volume of the series *The History of Sexuality: The Will to Knowledge* (1976). In this book, Foucault proposed that sexuality should no longer be regarded as a force of nature (the Freudian view of sexuality as drive, but also the causality between sex, gender, and desire), but as a discursive object, a cultural construction that changes over time and is inextricably bound up with power. Foucault discussed changes in the modern view of sexuality, especially highlighting the influence of new sciences like psychiatry and sexology, which replaced the religious view of non-procreative sexuality as sin, in defining 'normal' and 'abnormal' sexuality. The words 'heterosexuality' and 'homosexuality' were only coined by European physicians and psychiatrists in the last decades of the nineteenth century. They designed taxonomies based on sexual behaviour and desire. For example, the German-Austrian psychiatrist Richard von Krafft-Ebing (1840–1902) listed 'perversions' such as necrophilia, paedophilia, fetishism, sadism, and masochism in his famous book *Psychopathia Sexualis* (1886). The German physician Magnus Hirschfeld (1868–1935) wrote about transvestism, advocated gay and transgender rights, and founded the Institute for Sexology in Berlin in 1919.[31] This generation of psychiatrists and sexologists therefore balanced an interest in 'deviant' acts with compassion for people with non-mainstream desires and behaviour.

Foucault underlined that these academic 'descriptions' in fact also exerted power by dividing people into those with 'normal' and those with 'abnormal' sexualities. Moreover, the French philosopher argued that the discourses on modern sexuality were predicated on a notion of inner, individual identity. Whereas before the modern period, people might engage in same-sex sexual *acts*, in the modern period Foucault noted a shift from sexual acts to sexual *identity*. The homosexual became a persona with a specific identity derived from his or her sexual interests and activities, often including a deviant gender status, like an effeminate man.[32]

The field of the history of sexuality owes much to Foucault, since his work paved the way for studying sexuality as a cultural, and thus historically variable, construction. Nevertheless, not all historical work on sexuality or homosexuality is fully in accordance with Foucault's ideas. Firstly, the early books and articles on the history of homosexuality often aimed at providing a history of forefathers and foremothers. By excavating the presence of gay people in the past, the authors of these works not only underlined historical continuity, but also made an essentialist assumption that homosexuality was unchanging.[33] This type of 'gay history' does not dovetail with Foucault's notion of the differences between modern and premodern discourses on sexuality.

Secondly, many historians have accepted Foucault's suggestion of a shift from sexual acts between men or between women to a modern homosexual identity, but have located this shift in an earlier period than Foucault himself did. Theo van der Meer, for example, argues that a common understanding of the category of the 'sodomite' had emerged in western Europe by the late eighteenth century. This category was used both by homosexuals themselves and by the prosecutors and judges who indicted homosexuals, sodomy at the time being a capital crime. In the Netherlands, in the period before 1730, sodomy as a crime was kept quiet and prosecutions took place behind closed doors, but after the discovery and prosecution of numerous homosexual networks in 1730, a Foucauldian 'desire for knowledge' about homosexuality came into being. Publications and court records testify to an older notion of sodomy, namely as one of the many effects of gluttony, together with gambling and whoring. In this model, based on the early modern perception of the 'unruly' body, anyone could end up engaging in same-sex activity. Until circa 1675, the gay men prosecuted had often had sex of a hierarchical nature, with one man having an active role and the other, often a younger man, a passive role. From the last decades of the seventeenth century, however, van der Meer finds examples of adult men who alternated these roles and were often also part of a homosexual subculture:

> Participants in the subcultures met at public meeting sites or in private parlors, pubs and brothels; they had developed a bodily comportment – gestures and signals – and a slang that usually resembled those of prostitutes, who often picked up their customers at the same public sites. Effeminacy and camp-like behavior were rampant and some participants in these subcultures indulged in travesty.[34]

The prosecutions of 1730 led to a new categorization for men of what was permissible and impermissible sexual behaviour; sodomites were seen as 'effeminate'. The dualism between mind and body gave way to a unity in which desires were understood as being both mental and physical. Increasingly, homosexuals themselves felt part of a community of men who were the same and recognizable from the outside. They started to regard their feelings as innate and part of a homosexual self-awareness. Egalitarianism led not only to more equal marital relationships, but also to modern partner bonds between men. Thus, van der Meer argues that the shift to a homosexual identity, as identified by Foucault, did indeed take place, but a century earlier, and that it was not imposed by scientists, but rather grew up among administrators, commentators, and homosexuals themselves.[35]

▶ Queer theory and the body

Historians of sexuality have thus incorporated the idea, also presented by Foucault, that sexuality is a culturally variable organization of desire and sexual behaviour. This perspective is further theorized in queer studies, which branched off from gender studies in the 1990s and was strongly influenced by poststructuralist theory.[36] 'To queer' means to make strange, and queer studies intend to deconstruct natural assumptions on the entanglements of gender, sexuality, desire, and the body. 'Queer' is defined by queer theorist David Halperin as: *'whatever* is at odds with the normal, the legitimate, the dominant. *There is nothing in particular to which it necessarily refers*. It is an identity without an essence'. [37]

In her influential book *Gender Trouble* (1990), the philosopher Judith Butler, one of the foremost queer theorists, builds on the theories of scholars such as Georg Hegel, Sigmund Freud, Jacques Lacan, Michel Foucault, Jacques Derrida, Joan Riviere, and Simone de Beauvoir to argue that masculine or feminine behaviour (gender) does not naturally follow from being born with a male or female body (sex). Taking a drag queen (a male body dressing up as a woman) or a lesbian couple in which one woman displays more 'masculine' and the other more 'feminine' behaviour as examples that parody the 'normal' performance of gender and sexuality, Butler demonstrates the performativity of gender. Gender, that is, needs to be repeatedly performed in order to appear 'real'. A woman who puts on a dress and makeup every day performs 'femininity', thereby giving the impression that this behaviour follows naturally from having a female body. If we perform gender slightly differently, like the drag queen, Butler proposes, we can make 'gender trouble' and show that gendered behaviour is not natural but culturally constructed. Acts and bodily gestures which are learned and repeated over time, Butler explains,

> are *performative* in the sense that the essence or identity that they otherwise purport to express are *fabrications* manufactured and sustained through corporeal signs and discursive means. That the gendered body is performative suggests it has no ontological status apart from the various acts which constitute its reality.[38]

Butler argues that there is no initial core gendered body; this only acquires meaning during performative behaviour in society, when the person directs her/ his behaviour in line with cultural scripts about gender and (hetero)sexuality. By taking the cultural discourses as the starting point, and the body as a blank slate upon which these discourses work, Butler makes a radical stand in terms of social constructionism and builds on Foucault's view of sexuality as a 'fictitious unity between sex, gender and desire'[39]: 'The tactical production of the discrete and binary categorization of sex conceals the strategic aims of that very apparatus of production by postulating "sex" as "a cause" of sexual experience, behaviour, and desire.'[40]

Butler elaborates on the role of the body in these social processes of making meaning in her book *Bodies That Matter: On the Discursive Limits of 'Sex'* (1993), in which she discusses what counts as a body (and thus, which bodies *matter*). Again, in her account, the body is culturally constructed through language and performance.[41] She argues that cultural norms on gender and sexuality are so powerful that they discursively shape the body. Butler gives the example of a midwife who looks at the genitals of a newborn baby and concludes 'It's a girl.' For Butler this is a performative speech act: it is through the saying of these words that the baby is made into a girl. Western societies attach much value to genitals as the indicator of femaleness or maleness. However, we might envision it differently: why don't we classify newborn babies on the basis of other bodily features or simply refrain from bodily classification and call them 'babies'? Butler's aim is to denaturalize the purportedly biological statements that produce and maintain gender norms. Another example she gives is society's emphasis on the female body's capacity for impregnation as evidence of female bodily difference.[42] Butler points out that this description of women's bodies seems to describe biological reality, but in fact it assumes that only those bodies that can become pregnant count as female. In this, women who, for whatever reason, have not reproduced are not seen as 'real' women. Like Laqueur, Butler is keen to unmask biological statements as cultural ideas, which often discriminate against women or LGBTQ people. She asks 'under what discursive and institutional conditions, do certain biological differences ... become the salient characteristics of sex?'.[43]

On the one hand, Butler builds on de Beauvoir's argument that gender is shaped by culture, but on the other hand she rejects de Beauvoir's assumption of sex as biological and unchanging. For Butler both gender and sex are culturally constructed; indeed she reverses the commonly perceived causality between sex and gender (the sexed body determining gendered behaviour) and argues, similarly to Laqueur, that we read sex through the lens of gender. Some critics have interpreted Butler's rejection of the sex–gender distinction as a complete dismissal of sex, and thus of the body. However, as Samuel Chambers argues, 'Butler does not maintain the thesis that sex is nothing more than gender, and she certainly does not reject, deny, elide or erase the body'.[44] Other critics have found fault with the lack of space for individual, bodily agency within her position of discursive constructionism.[45] These objections are discussed in Chapter 6 on new materialism.

Generally, queer theory has opened up the field of sexuality studies, by addressing homosexuality, heterosexuality, transgender,[46] and other aspects of sexuality. The term 'queer' has an open meaning, potentially including every type of sexual behaviour. This 'celebration of ambiguous and non-unified subject positions',[47] derived from its poststructuralist emphasis on the (discursive) construction of identity, has also been criticized by gay and transgender scholars and readers. Some of them fear that the activist part of sexuality studies and the history of sexuality may be lost because homosexuals or transgender people are no longer defined as having a fixed identity, which makes it harder to campaign for social change or gay and transgender liberation on the basis of a common identity.[48] Moreover, especially in the case of transgender people, the wish to have a 'real' material female or male body, rather than to belong to a fluid category, can sit uneasily with queer theory.[49]

Many of the claims presented by queer theorists dovetail with the findings of historians of sexuality. Both historians of sexuality and queer theorists explore the historically and culturally variable relationships between body, gender, and desire. This includes studying heterosexuality as a cultural construction,[50] but also debates on the continuities and change in the history of lesbianism and intersex people.[51] These histories thus 'queer' the relationships between sex, gender, and the self.

▷ The western-centrism of histories of gender and sexuality

These historically shifting conceptions of the sexed body have to take into account more than gender and sexuality. Therefore, historian Jeanne Boydston criticizes gender historians for applying gender as a rigid category: for taking their starting point in present-day western gender binaries and projecting these onto the past, but also for not paying enough attention to the ways the category of gender intersects with other identity categories such as race, class, age, and sexuality. Boydston builds on the work of a number of non-western historians who claim that not all societies were organized along the male-female binary.[52] The African historian Oyèrónké Oyewúmí, for instance, argues that western work on gender has been preoccupied with two oppositionally sexed bodies, which invests the category 'gender' with a rigid corporeal determinism. Underlining the historically specific valorization of the body, Oyewúmí regards the two-sexed binary as Euro- and western-centric. In pre-colonial Yoruba culture, Oyewúmí points out, the *primary* principle of social classification was seniority, rather than gender.[53]

Similarly, the primacy of the male-female binary can be problematized by taking into account the presence of 'third' or 'fourth' genders in Native American cultures (female-sexed persons who performed 'male' social and economic roles, and vice versa). The idea that some people did not fit into the categories of male and female and therefore inhabited a 'third sex' is found in many countries and in different periods. It surfaces in the term 'berdache', which was coined by French explorers, traders, and missionaries in the seventeenth and eighteenth centuries who encountered Native Americans not conforming with European gender classifications: these included males who did women's work, wore women's clothing, combined men's and women's attire, or had relationships with non-berdache men. 'Berdache' was a pejorative term, to classify deviant behaviour, which is why since 1990 researchers have put forward other terms for this tradition, such as 'two-spirit'.[54] Research into tribes that considered two-spirit people normal is seen by some historians as an opportunity to loosen the association between gender and (two-sex, reproductive) bodies. Moreover, in indigenous cultures the female–male binary was probably no more important than other binaries such as war–peace, young–old, plant–animal, etc.[55]

Since the association with male and female reproductive bodies haunts the concept of gender, Boydston suggests historians focus on 'historically grounded histories of particular processes of gendering, resulting in distinct cultural meanings with distinct social and cultural formations – gender, that is to say, as cultural process, various and altering over time (even within the modern period and even within western culture)'.[56] Boydston here, from the perspective of gender history, reaches a similar conclusion to that put forward by queer scholars: that the relationship between body and gender is culturally variable.

▷ Conclusion

This chapter has tried to disentangle the relationships between the body, gender, and desire. We have seen how both historians and queer theorists have deconstructed ideas on the naturalness of the existence of two sexes, which supposedly determine gendered behaviour and sexual desire. This deconstruction can firstly be achieved by demonstrating how the markers of femininity and masculinity – varying from genitals, to gonads, hormones, and chromosomes – shift over time. Moreover, the historian Laqueur and the philosophers Foucault and Butler especially have shown how bodily sex and sexuality are also cultural constructs, although it is not always completely clear how sex and gender relate to one another. For the philosopher de Beauvoir the female body was mostly negative, and she focused on the cultural construction of gender, rather than the body. Gender historians in the 1980s also assumed that gender was more important than physical sexual distinctions. Laqueur brought the body back onto the historical scene: he too viewed it through the social-constructionist lens. However, gender remained the primary viewpoint, since Laqueur argued that ideas on masculinity and femininity, as formulated for instance in humoral theory, determined the position of the body in the cultural imagination.

Adding to the argument that the body is culturally constructed, Butler put forward the idea that gendered behaviour needs to be performed in order to convey the impression of reality. She thus inserted the body into the performance of gender and sexuality. Where for Laqueur gender norms were primary and determined the perception of the sexed body, Butler suggested that the heterosexual norm forcefully shaped gendered behaviour.

Apart from the objection that these theorists of gender and sexuality often neglect other axes of identity such as ethnicity, race, or age, another point of criticism aimed at theorists like Foucault and Butler is that they focus too much on powerful discourses on the body, gender, and sexuality, rather than on individual experiences of the material body. In particular, some scholars have wondered whether these discourses are as powerful as discursive constructionists would have us believe. The historian Ivan Crozier, for example, argues that historians, in focusing on sexological discourse about 'perversions' such as 'the homosexual' or the 'sadomasochist', have a tendency to equate sexual acts with sexual identities, instead of investigating the actual use of bodies and their experience of pleasure.[57] In fact, Crozier states, homosexuals have reacted to their medicalization in different ways: by criticizing it, accepting it, or ignoring it.[58]

To summarize, although in the works of poststructuralist thinkers like Foucault and Butler agency is often found to be lacking, it is generally accepted that these authors have contributed to unmasking the seemingly natural categories of sex and gender as culturally constructed, and to problematizing the relationships between sex, gender, and desire. Historians, however, have been the ones to demonstrate the potential of these theories by providing examples of the historically variable constructions of sex and gender.

5 Experiencing the Body

▶ Introduction

The previous two chapters discussed scholars, such as Foucault and Butler, who emphasize how the body is given meaning through **discourse**. These approaches have been a helpful correction to naturalistic essentialism by shifting our attention to cultural constructions of the body and gender; however, they often limit the meaning of bodies to being symbolic and discursive signifiers, to the neglect of the material and lived experience, or the phenomenology, of the body.[1] This chapter provides an overview of different theories that highlight the body as experienced by individuals. The central notion here is the term 'embodiment', which is here defined as the 'lived body'. It is comparable to the German *Leib*, which refers to the living, felt body, whereas *Körper* denotes the body as object. The concept of the lived body rejects Cartesian dualism, which rigidly separates mind from body and regards the body as a material object. The lived body is directed towards relationships with other people, other things, and the environment and is thus bound up with an experienced world.[2]

Sociologists have pointed out that embodiment involves social processes: body techniques like walking and dancing need to be learned in a social context and in relation to other people. Bryan Turner highlights three aspects of embodiment: 'having a body in which the body has the characteristics of a thing, being a body in which we are subjectively engaged with our body as a project, and doing a body in the sense of producing a body through time'.[3] Cultural historians have used the notion of embodiment to include both cultural norms of the body, and the ways individuals incorporate or reject those norms. The historian Kathleen Canning regards the notion of embodiment, which approaches bodily practices as contextual, as 'a far less fixed and idealised concept than body', encompassing 'moments of encounter and interpretation, agency and resistance'.[4] The concept of embodiment here functions as a bridge between seeing the body as purely constructed by cultural norms and taking the individual body as an unproblematic source of experience.

It is only since the 1960s that social scientists, and later historians, have started to shift their attention from institutions to personal interactions. In medical sociology, the patient's experience and subjectivity came to the fore, in the use of the term 'illness narratives', or the ways in which patients described their illnesses, including metaphors, cognitive representations, and images.[5] Historians of medicine, too, became interested in what Roy Porter called 'the patient's point of view',[6] stimulating publications on the social history of health and disease from the perspective of historical individuals. In the late 1980s and 1990s, however, poststructuralist historians questioned to what extent a 'real' experience could be retrieved, since experiences are constructed by culture and language. Joan Scott argued that historians of gender and homosexuality, keen to make the lives of forgotten men and women visible, had too often accepted the experience found for instance in autobiographical writing of women or homosexuals as directly and unproblematically shaping their identities, which thus became self-evident rather than historically variable. Instead of taking experience as evidence of historical fact, Scott encouraged historians to critically study the notion of 'experience' itself.[7]

This chapter discusses different theoretical approaches that all attempt to lay bare individual bodily experiences. It firstly considers the most influential set of theories in relation to the lived body: phenomenology, a branch of philosophy here represented by the French philosopher Maurice Merleau-Ponty. This section includes critical perspectives on phenomenology, as found especially in the works of psychiatrist and political activist Frantz Fanon, and philosopher Iris Marion Young, who added the racial and gendered experiences of the body to the more universal phenomenological approach of Merleau-Ponty. Secondly, the chapter discusses 'historical phenomenology', the application of insights from phenomenology by historians and literary scholars. So far, historians have not drawn on phenomenology very often, instead applying Bourdieu's notion of 'habitus', which also highlights the social components of the lived body. Therefore, the third part of this chapter critically examines how Bourdieu's insights have been used by historians of the body and emotions. Last, given that phenomenological approaches have been criticized for not being able to accurately reconstruct individual bodily experiences, this chapter briefly investigates to what extent historians can use psychoanalytical concepts, including attention for the unconscious, to make sense of bodily experience.

▶ Phenomenology

Phenomenology is the branch of philosophy that studies the structures of consciousness as experienced from the first-person point of view. It addresses the meanings things have in our experience, including aspects such as perception, thought, memory, imagination, emotion, desire, volition, bodily awareness, embodied action, and social activity. Phenomenology pays attention to how objects, events, the self, and time are actively and passively experienced to form our 'life world'. The body is central to this experience. Phenomenologists have included the twentieth-century philosophers Edmund Husserl, Martin Heidegger, Jean-Paul Sartre, and Simone de Beauvoir.

In 1940s Paris, Maurice Merleau-Ponty (1908–1961) joined the existentialist philosophers Sartre and de Beauvoir in developing phenomenology. They were interested in a concrete philosophy of daily life, in contrast to the reigning intellectualist and rationalist philosophy of the time.[8] In *Phenomenology of Perception* (1945) Merleau-Ponty emphasizes the role of the body in human experience and focuses on the 'body image', our experience of our own body and its significance in our activities. Merleau-Ponty thus resists the traditional Cartesian separation of mind and body, making the body the primary site of knowing the world and locating subjectivity in the body, instead of in mind and consciousness. For Merleau-Ponty, our bodies are our way of being-in-the-world.[9] The body is thus no longer an object, but a body subject.[10]

Merleau-Ponty rejects the dichotomous divisions of inner and outer, subject and object that characterize much of modern philosophy. He gives the example of a person whose right hand touches his or her left hand, causing the double sensation of being both (a touching) subject and (a touched) object.[11] In being at the same time perceiver and perceived, the lived body is an 'intertwining',[12] and experience is therefore located midway between mind and body.[13] For Merleau-Ponty, consciousness – an active attitude directed towards things, rather than a passive substance – is intentional and embodied (in the world), and equally the body is infused with consciousness (cognition of the world).[14] As Merleau-Ponty explains:

> We grasp external space through our bodily situation. A 'corporeal or postural schema' gives us at every moment a global, practical, and implicit notion of the relation between our body and things, of our hold on them. A system of possible movements, or 'motor projects,' radiates from us to our environment. Our body is not in space like things; it inhabits or haunts space. It applies itself to space like

a hand to an instrument, and when we wish to move about we do not move the body as we move an object. We transport it without instruments as if by magic, since it is ours and because through it we have direct access to space. For us the body [...] is our expression in the world, the visible form of our intentions.[15]

The refreshing attention for corporeal experience has appealed to other scholars, but they have also criticized Merleau-Ponty's thinking for being too universal. Iris Marion Young has taken up his phenomenology from a feminist perspective, and Frantz Fanon from a postcolonial perspective.

▶ Feminist critique of phenomenology: Iris Marion Young

Feminist philosopher Iris Marion Young (1949–2006) built on the insights of phenomenologist philosophers Merleau-Ponty and de Beauvoir in her article 'Throwing like a Girl; A Phenomenology of Feminine Body Comportment Motility and Spatiality' (1980). Merleau-Ponty claimed that the relation of a subject to its world was defined by the purposive orientation of the body towards the world surrounding this subject. The intentional moves that a body makes constitute the possibilities for the subject that are opened up in the world. De Beauvoir, however, had argued that women, as the Other, were not able to develop their subjectivity because of the particular, discriminating, situation they found themselves in. Young also took on this idea of the inhibiting situation for women.

Young observed that women often do not make full use of the space around them: men are more open in their gait and stride, swinging their arms, whereas women tend to keep their legs together when sitting and to hold their arms across their bodies. While women carry their books close to their chests, boys and men swing them along their sides. Women experience the space surrounding them as a constricting space:

> Not only is there a typical style of throwing like a girl, but there is a more or less typical style of running like a girl, climbing like a girl, swinging like a girl, hitting like a girl. They have in common, first, that the whole body is not put into fluid and directed motion, but rather, in swinging and hitting for example, the motion is concentrated in one body part; and second, that the woman's motin [sic] tends not to reach, extend, lean, stretch and follow through in the direction of her intention.[16]

Young concludes that feminine movement is hallmarked by 'ambiguous transcendence, inhibited intentionality, and a discontinuous unity with its surroundings'.[17] Whereas for Merleau-Ponty, the body is a subject, for women, Young argues, the body is experienced as both subject and object. Women do not always feel in control of their bodies and are uncertain of their movements, their bodies functioning as objects rather than originators of motion. Thus, 'the modalities of feminine bodily comportment ... have their source in the particular *situation* of women as conditioned by their sexist oppression in contemporary society.'[18] Women's inhibition and protection of their bodies might, according to Young, also stem from a defence against bodily invasion, since women often encounter unsafe environments. Young therefore unmasks Merleau-Ponty's bodily subject as implicitly masculine. These universalist assumptions have also been criticized from a postcolonialist perspective by Frantz Fanon.

▶ Postcolonial critique of phenomenology: Frantz Fanon

The postcolonial work of Frantz Fanon (1925–1961) reveals influences of Sartre's existentialist thought, (Freudian and Lacanian) psychoanalysis, and phenomenology.[19] Born in the French colony of Martinique, Fanon was one of the few black children who could study at the lycée and he thought of himself as French. When he joined the French army in 1944, he experienced racism from his fellow soldiers and from the French population. After the war, Fanon studied medicine in France, eventually specializing in psychiatry, and later worked as a psychiatrist in Algeria.[20] In his work, particularly in his book *Black Skin, White Masks* (1952), Fanon describes and analyzes the mental and bodily experience of being a black man in a colonial world. Particularly in France, Fanon experienced an otherness as a black man, feeling the weight of the 'white gaze'. In a train in France, a white girl pointed to him calling out, 'Look, a negro!'. At that moment, Fanon describes, his image of his body changed and fell apart:

> I was responsible not only for my body but also for my race and my ancestors. I cast an objective gaze over myself, discovered my blackness, my ethnic features; deafened by cannibalism, backwardness, fetishism, racial stigmas, slave traders, [...] Disoriented, incapable of confronting the Other, the white man, who had no scruples about imprisoning me, I transported myself on that particular day far, very far, from my self, and gave myself up as an object. What did this mean to

me? Peeling, stripping my skin, causing a hemorrhage that left congealed black blood all over my body. Yet this reconsideration of myself, this thematization, was not my idea. I wanted simply to be a man among men.[21]

As Fanon argues, it is only in the encounter with the white imagination that a phenomenology of blackness – the experience of skin difference and of being the black Other – becomes manifest. This includes a historical burden of slavery and stereotypes of black people, which the white imagination imposes on the black man and which is internalized by him. Fanon writes, 'I am overdetermined from the outside. [...] The white gaze, the only valid one, is already dissecting me. I am *fixed*. Once their microtomes are sharpened, the Whites objectively cut sections of my reality.'[22]

Fanon uses Merleau-Ponty's emphasis on bodily experience to account for racial identity formation. But he is also critical of Merleau-Ponty's notion of the 'corporeal schema', which assumes the body's free agency to actively perceive the surrounding world. Fanon, however, points out that this does not automatically apply to the black man. He quotes Merleau-Ponty and at the same time criticizes his insights:

> Beneath the body schema I had created a historical-racial schema. The data I used were provided not by 'remnants of feelings and notions of the tactile, vestibular, kinesthetic, or visual nature,' but by the Other, the white man, who had woven me out of a thousand details, anecdotes, and stories.[23]

Fanon replaces Merleau-Ponty's notion of the 'corporeal schema' first with the 'historico-racial schema' and then with the 'racial epidermal schema'. The free movement of the perceiving body, as envisioned by Merleau-Ponty, is prevented first by history, as constructed by a white imagery that is cast upon the black subject, and second by the fixation of the white gaze on the black subject's body, accentuating black skin as the defining characteristic of the black subject.[24] The body is thus *made* black.[25] For Fanon, white people are able to participate in the schematization of the world, but black people in the interracial encounter do not have this free agency. Merleau-Ponty's inclusive, universal rendering of the corporeal schema cannot be applied in a colonized and racially oppressive world. The black person's bodily comportment – for instance in deciding whether or not to make eye contact with the white person – must be scrutinized constantly so as not to overstep the invisible racial boundaries.[26] Whereas classical phenomenology assumes the ability to move independently, Fanon's phenomenology of the black body stresses an experience of restriction.[27] The black man is prevented from becoming a full bodily subject, he experiences the consciousness of his body as 'third person consciousness', as an amputation.[28]

Fanon's work on black embodiment is powerful for several reasons. Firstly, he shows how racial identity is formed in and on the body and acknowledges that this is a traumatic experience, which reveals that Fanon was influenced not only by phenomenology, but also by psychoanalytical notions. The split identification known from psychoanalysis, which emphasized difference and otherness *within* the self, dovetails with Fanon's description of the formation of black identity.[29]

Secondly, Fanon contests the view that essentialism, and in particular black essentialism, is based on biology.[30] At the time of writing, 1952, this was by no means a common opinion. Dismantling phenomenology's universalism, Fanon presents us with the (colonial) reality in which embodiment is experienced differently by black and white people,[31] in this way also demonstrating the cultural variability of the lived body. Phenomenology may therefore help us make aware that whiteness is an effect of racialization.[32] More generally, a phenomenological approach can reveal how individuals take on race-conscious habitual postures; this approach demonstrates how cultural conceptions of race work in corporeal behaviour on a micro-level.[33]

▷ History of bodily experience: Barbara Duden

Phenomenology is one of the few theoretical approaches that accords a central place to the body; nevertheless, it has not often been applied by historians. In the following sections, I present a number of scholars who have used insights from phenomenology in an attempt to access the (bodily) experience of people in the past.

One of the first books in body history that was keen to reconstruct bodily experience was Barbara Duden's *The Woman Beneath the Skin. A Doctor's Patients in Eighteenth-Century Germany* (1987), in which she noted that historians had failed to take corporeal experiences seriously:

> Scholars study the physical conditions of people in the past and examine patterns of fertility, birth practices, nursing habits, and the frequency of intercourse in different historical cultures. But what people in a different age and culture

thought about the inside of the body, about the hidden sphere under the skin, about stomach, breast, blood, and excrement, about the 'life inside the body,' is virtually unknown and rarely looked at.[34]

Duden studied more than 1800 case histories noted down by the German doctor Johannes Pelargius Storch around 1730, including female patients' letters to him. In their letters to Dr Storch, these German women described the movements of their bodies, perceived via sensations and understood via analogies linking these different perceptions. This early modern body had a number of characteristics: it was seen as permeable via different orifices and the skin, as internally undifferentiated, and as strongly interactive with the environment; sex differences were negligible, and the body was not yet measured against a norm of health or illness as in modernity. Duden writes: 'The female body implied in Storch's accounts is not a visible object which takes up space and within which its organs are located. The blood embodied in the women is more like an orientational surge, creating space as it flows.'[35] Duden traces a shift from an early modern sensation-based bodily self-knowledge, in which women were the authorities on their own bodies, to a modern, visually directed, bodily self-knowledge, in which the body is an object looked at from the outside by (male) medical experts with the help of medical technology like a microscope or ultrasound. Duden thus argues that there was a vast difference between early modern and modern bodily experience. The modern 'interiorless' self, read from the outside by medical experts, in this reading becomes less authentic and less autonomous than the early modern bodily experience.[36]

Duden was influenced by several kinds of phenomenological analyses of the body as an object of perception.[37] She combines her phenomenological approach with a 'method of self-reflexive, scrupulous historicism',[38] distancing herself from her own views on the body (and thus from her own body): the modern definition of the body as a stable anatomico-physiological collection of organs. She tried to retain a sense of alienation, an awareness of the strangeness of these early modern stories of the body.[39] Writing before the linguistic turn, Duden pays scant attention to the role of language and text, and her analysis has also been criticized for presenting the popular bodily experience as initially unchanging and then suddenly devoured by the rising academic discipline of medicine at the start of the nineteenth century. In addition, questions have been raised about her portrayal of the early modern bodily self as more authentic and thus immune to cultural construction.[40] However, Duden's book remains one of the most successful attempts to get at the historical experience of the body, because it is based on first-person experiences that are explained with reference to the cultural context.

▶ Historical phenomenology: The passions

Given the 'otherness' of the early modern body, it is perhaps no surprise that phenomenological approaches to the body have been applied most often by historians of the early modern period, especially by a number of literary scholars who study early modern drama. It was in this field that the notion of 'historical phenomenology'[41] was coined, at the intersection of sensory history, the history of emotion, and the affective turn within the social sciences. Focusing on relationships and the troubling boundaries between intrinsic and extrinsic, subject and object, historical phenomenology is described as embracing 'the dynamism and nebulousness of feeling and sensation by thinking in terms of ecologies rather than artifacts [sic], experiences rather than objects, and by abandoning net distinctions between persons and things.'[42]

One example of the application of historical phenomenology in the field of early modern drama studies is the work by Gail Kern Paster, *Humoring the Body: Emotions and the Shakespearean Stage* (2010). In her book, Paster distinguishes between on the one hand pre-Enlightenment emotions – determined by humoral theory, part of the fabric of the porous and volatile body, and connected to the environment – and on the other hand modern emotions, which were part of the solid body. What we moderns consider emotional figuration, Paster argues, was for early modern people often a bodily reality: spleens were seen as producing melancholy, and the size of livers and gall bladders was thought to determine boldness; melancholy was not *caused* by black bile, but literally resided in it.[43] In the Galenic scheme of the six non-naturals, the passions (together with air, diet, repletion, evacuation, sleep, and exercise) determined bodily well-being. Like the humours, the passions were thought to run through the blood stream, carrying blood, phlegm, choler, and melancholy: 'For the early moderns, the power of the passions was a function of the affect-producing organs – the blood-making liver, the hungry heart, the angry gall bladder, and the melancholy spleen'.[44]

Paster aims to find out what passions felt like in this type of body, hence her interest in the phenomenological character of early modern emotions. Taking from Merleau-Ponty an interest in the individual subject's phenomenological

experience in relation to the social field,[45] Paster posits an 'ecology of the passions' to emphasize that the environment directly interacts with the emotions: for
instance winds were metaphorically described as passions: the passions were 'the
winds and the waves of the body', and the body was filled with moving currents
of air in the bloodstream. Similarly, it was believed that the devil, since he inhabited the air, could be inhaled into the bloodstream and could thus be given the
opportunity to infect people's hearts and minds.[46] A phenomenological approach
thus allows Paster to reconstruct the bodily experience of the passions in the early
modern period, including its relationship with the outer environment. However,
since her work is based on the study of Shakespeare's plays, contextualized by
early modern medical texts, moral treatises, natural history accounts, and other
literary texts, one might wonder how the *representation* of corporeal experience in
these sources relates to the understanding of the passions in daily life.

▶ Historical phenomenology: Pain

This relationship between the lived body and its representation in text or images
is a complex one, and one of the most persistent problems for writing body history. The difficulty comes to the fore particularly in the historiography of pain.
Pain is one of the central notions when it comes to rendering the experience of
the human body. Historians have raised the question how we can reconstruct
and interpret the experience of pain in the past and, more generally, how we can
'grasp the body as perceived subjectively, from the inside'.[47] A major obstacle in
this endeavour is that historians have to rely mainly on written sources, and it is
doubtful whether the expression of pain on paper accurately reflects the feeling
itself. In short, the history of pain raises the problem of the relationship between
feeling and language.

Literary scholar Elaine Scarry, in her book *The Body in Pain* (1985), argues that
pain is outside language, private and untransmittable. Historian Joanna Bourke
refutes this position, stating that it reifies pain, and that by making pain an independent agent Scarry has fallen into the 'ontological trap' of taking metaphorical
descriptions of pain as descriptions of an actual entity.[48] Bourke wants to conceive of pain as a life event, a way of perceiving an experience. Regarding pain as
'a way of being-in-the-world' implies that people 'do' pain, they construct pain.[49]
Conceiving pain as an event allows Bourke to highlight that pain can be affected
by environmental interactions, as well as by interactions with other persons, and

that it can be learned and communicated, and is thus social. Bourke also emphasizes that the act of naming influences bodily responses, thereby breaking down
the dichotomy between body and mind.[50]

Bourke's view of pain as 'a way of being-in-the-world' dovetails with the
phenomenological emphasis on lived experience and embodied consciousness.[51] She underlines the interconnections between language, culture, and the
body, assuming that bodies are actively engaged in constructing the experience of pain: 'autonomic arousal, cardiovascular responses, and sensorimotor
actions influence the way people think: the body provides possibilities (and
constraints) for the metaphors adopted'.[52] She builds on the work of cognitive
linguists, who state that people construct image schemata from sensorimotor
corporeal experiences, which are then projected onto the wider world via metaphors. Bourke, however, claims that these image schemata are not universal but
historically changing. For example, in the eighteenth century the metaphors
used to describe the body stemmed from humoral theory, in which pain was
regarded as the result of an imbalance. In this model, the body was continually
in flux (rather than a separate entity distinguished from the mind, as in the later
twentieth-century biomedical model) and pain – or the blockage of natural flows
– circulated in the whole body.[53] Bourke concludes that 'eighteenth-century bod-
ies-in-pain *felt* different to modern ones. The figurative languages of humoral
bodies reveal different ways of being-in-the world'.[54] She shows how pain metaphors were drawn from everyday encounters. For instance, the construction of
railways in the mid-nineteenth century impacted directly on the metaphorical
language of pain, including the imagery of arteries as railway tracks and throb-
bing inflammations as railway engines. Similarly, electricity featured widely in
pain metaphors from the early nineteenth century. During the industrial age the
humoral metaphors started to disappear, and pain was decreasingly depicted as
a demon.[55]

In this phenomenological approach, social and environmental interactions
help *create* the body (rather than merely *representing* the body); the body and
the social world mutually constitute each other. For Bourke, this approach has
a number of advantages: it problematizes body-mind dualism, it makes possible
the study of different bodies, and it provides an opportunity to explore the ways
sensations change over time.[56] Her approach to the history of pain, especially
the focus on cultural metaphors, also takes into account cultural and historical
variability, as well as a collective bodily experience. To a lesser extent, however,
it discusses individual feelings of pain.

▶ Historical phenomenology: Race

Let us delve deeper into this relationship between individual bodily experience and its representation in cultural discourses and texts. How have other scholars applied phenomenological insights in interpreting this relationship? While Duden used eighteenth-century doctor-patient correspondence and Paster early modern plays, literary scholar Katherine Fishburn chose nineteenth-century African-American slave narratives to study embodiment in relation to race. Issues of body and mind are regular elements in African-American slave narratives, which were written to highlight the humanity and civil rights of this group. In thus acknowledging African Americans' minds and intellects, the narratives clashed with the association, common in nineteenth-century American culture, between black people and the body. Arguably, these slave narratives thus display a tension between the body as marker of self-identification and the body as object of (white) violence.[57] A phenomenological approach, however, can overcome the body-mind dichotomy, which in this case is conflated with ideas on race. Fishburn applies a phenomenological reading to argue that 'Rather than seeing the ex-slaves' embodiment as something to be denied, underplayed, or overcome, I began to see it as the route to a new kind of knowing – one based in the body, or, as I prefer to call it, one based in the body-self.'[58] Unlike white people, the slaves did not have the luxury of forgetting their bodies. In their description of gestures, labouring, singing, dancing, and walking, Fishburn argues, they 'used the gift of their embodiment to … redefine what it means to be human'.[59]

In addition to connecting body and mind, Fishburn follows Merleau-Ponty in demonstrating the interconnectedness people experience through their bodies. When, for instance, formerly enslaved author Frederick Douglass (1818–1895), in his *Narrative of the Life of Frederick Douglass, an American Slave. Written by Himself* (1845), writes about how as a young boy he witnessed his Aunt Hester being cruelly beaten, this is the start of his own body turning into a slave's body. Fishburn argues that 'his body is learning its vulnerability and debasement at the hands of these other, more powerful, embodied beings and that his body is recognizing, for the first time, his connectedness to the other plantation slaves'.[60] Moreover, Douglass feels the pain of enslavement when he hears slave songs on the plantation, which greatly move him. Fishburn underlines that Douglass comes to understand the meaning of these songs – and thus of slavery – by seeing and hearing with his body.[61] In this study of the history of race, phenomenology can help overcome the body-mind division and emphasize the relationships between people, facilitated by bodily sympathy. However, it is also clear that these experiences are strongly determined by the genre of the African-American slave narrative, and that this in turn was influenced by the tradition of the American sentimental novel, in which the goal was to attain the readers' sympathy.[62] This fact does not make the corporeal experiences less 'real', but it does mean that textual mediation cannot be neglected.

▷ Bourdieu's notion of habitus

Apart from the phenomenological cue provided by Merleau-Ponty, many historians have also incorporated the notion of 'habitus' into their research to do justice to the role of the body; in this, they mainly used the term as applied by the French sociologist Pierre Bourdieu. I first outline Bourdieu's notion of habitus and then present examples of the way this concept has been applied by historians.

Bourdieu was not the first scholar to refer to 'habitus'. The French anthropologist Marcel Mauss (1872–1950) already spoke of 'techniques of the body' in a lecture in 1935, in which he asked how different societies could have different corporeal habits, varying from different swimming techniques to different postures for sleeping. These techniques of the body, which vary according to sex, age, and culture, are learned behaviours: Mauss stresses socialization and education.[63] Mauss used the term 'habitus', which was later adopted by the French sociologist Pierre Bourdieu (1930–2002).

Bourdieu was interested in culture as 'practice', looking at the ways cultural ideas were inherited and performed, and how the family and the education system socialized children into replicating class- and gender-specific behaviour. He aimed at finding a middle way between regarding culture as an unchanging structure – imposed from above – and individual agency. Whereas 'objectivism' neglected the individual's actions, Bourdieu criticized phenomenology as an example of 'subjectivism', which in his view failed to note that lived experience was produced by the internalization of cultural and social structures. This might be regarded as a misreading of phenomenology, which does not restrict its inquiry to a description of the life world, but allows room for its connection to underlying structures. Moreover, Bourdieu's work often draws on phenomenological perspectives and can be regarded as overlapping with them.[64]

In applying the notion of 'habitus' Bourdieu, who was influenced by Merleau-Ponty as well as Goffman and Lévi-Strauss, strove to give room to both structure and agency and to give space to the body. Bourdieu defined habitus as the system of 'durable, transposable dispositions...which generate and organize practices and representations that can be objectively adapted to their outcomes without presupposing a conscious aiming at ends or an express mastery of the operations necessary in order to attain them'.[65] A bourgeois habitus, for example, may refer to the way children and later adults learn to incorporate class norms on etiquette by displaying the 'right' bodily posture and table manners. This learned behaviour becomes natural, 'second nature'. Habitus might also be defined as: 'embodied sensibility that makes possible structured improvisation'.[66] Bourdieu's attention to both the pre-reflexive and the learned character of our bodily automatisms reveals the influence of phenomenology.[67] Generally, structuration theories like Bourdieu's can be seen as providing a middle way between social-constructionist accounts of discipline and governmentality and a phenomenological emphasis on lived experience.[68] Although scholars differ in their interpretations of the habitus, emphasizing either the side of individual agency or the side of imposed structure,[69] the notion of habitus has been influential among cultural historians interested in the body.

The first example of this use of habitus comes from the field of the history of emotion. Historians have pointed out that emotions are not universal but vary across cultures and periods. However, they differ in their answers to the question how we can define emotions in the past: Are emotions cognitive or bodily? And can historians ever trace emotions as they were actually felt in the past? It has turned out to be easier to reconstruct cultural rules on emotions than the emotions themselves. Often historians assumed that the *experience* of emotions was universal, but their *expression* culturally variable. This assumption, however, artificially separates experience and expression, whereas these are often mutually influential. Historians are also forced to focus on written sources, and hence tend to study verbal expressions of emotions. As the historian Barbara Rosenwein states, this may lead to a neglect of non-verbal forms of emotional expression. For example, medieval Icelandic culture attached more value to blushing, swelling, and shaking than to a rendition of affect in words.[70] Increasingly, therefore, historians are trying to take into account the body in their research on emotions and the senses (sight, smell, touch, hearing, and taste).[71]

Historical and cultural anthropologist Monique Scheer, for instance, aims to include the body in her notion of 'emotional practices'. Trying to overcome a body–mind dualism, including a separation between the inner experience of emotions and their outer expression, Scheer studies emotion as a type of learned, embodied practice, building on Bourdieu's notion of habitus.[72] Scheer looks, for example, at emotional practices aimed at mobilizing emotions, such as court-ship rituals, which vary throughout history and 'serve to cultivate a certain kind of feeling between potential marriage partners – which can range from duti-ful obedience, to honor, to passion, admiration, familiarity, or respect'. In this view, courtship has 'performative effects on the constitution of feelings and the (gendered) self'.[73] This methodological focus on the situated 'doing' of emotions still relies on texts to trace observable actions, but is not, according to Scheer, limited to first-person accounts. Scheer suggests searching for language that links the body with the mind, which will probably go together with shifts in bodily practices: she gives the example of an increase in talk about 'interiority' being accompanied by the creation of private spaces.[74] In short, Bourdieu's notion of habitus paves the way for Scheer to study emotion as an embodied practice.

Another example of the application of Bourdieu's notion of habitus by historians is Herman Roodenburg's study of gesture in the early modern Dutch Republic. Since the Renaissance, higher-class persons were encouraged to 'fash-ion' and 'cultivate' their bodies. Manuals of civility, such as Erasmus' *De Civilitate Morum Puerilium* (1530) and Castiglione's *Il Libro del Cortegiano* (1528), which were reprinted and translated over and over, instructed the elite, especially its children, how to comport their bodies. In advice on standing, walking, sitting, fencing, dancing, and riding, the general recommendation was to have a nat-ural, elegant, and straight posture and a pleasing self-presentation. According to Dutch poet and composer Constantijn Huygens (1596–1687), his father was convinced that 'in the same way that the mind is formed by exercises, so the bodies of well-to-do children should learn to move in a dignified and elegant way'.[75] In this way, a focus on bodily habits demonstrates how (elite) norms and behaviour are passed on from generation to generation.

Roodenburg builds on Bourdieu's notions of habitus, the durable dispositions of all kinds of movements, and especially of those bodily automatisms which are part of the habitus and which Bourdieu defined as 'hexis'. Roodenburg also refers to the social anthropologist Paul Connerton,[76] who used the notion of 'bodily memory', the ways in which our bodies remember a certain performance, for instance when children are socialized into having a self-assured, upright bearing.[77] In Roodenburg's view, Bourdieu's concept of habitus has the disad-vantage of being passive, of something exposed from the outside, and of lacking historicity, since it is directed towards reproduction and continuity. For this reason, Roodenburg, following Connerton, prefers the notions of body memory or habitual memory to refer to habitual skills and bodily automatisms, since these notions highlight the active exercise needed.[78] However, other scholars regard Bourdieu's concept of habitus as dynamic, offering a good explanation for both the durability and the changeability of identity, and providing more room for material embodiment and for temporality.[79] Nevertheless, some critics have objected that even Bourdieu's notion of habitus offers little room for a phenomenological understanding of the lived body.[80] Therefore, in the final section of this chapter we turn to psychoanalytical theories, which claim to pay more attention to the inner, mental aspects of (bodily) experience.

▶ Psychoanalysis and the body in history

We have seen so far that phenomenological approaches, mostly deriving from the work of Merleau-Ponty, and Bourdieu's notion of habitus provide historians with instruments to assess bodily experience in the past. Another way for historians to interpret subjective corporeal experiences is to use concepts from psychoanalysis. Sigmund Freud's (1856–1939) psychoanalysis, developed from the 1890s onwards, accorded a central role to the unconscious, in particular unconscious human drives, such as sexual urges and aggression. Freud's model of the personality explained the human mind as consisting of ego, id, and super-ego: three contrasting elements, the id representing human drives, the super-ego the fatherly and cultural norms mostly forbidding these drives, and the ego that which is conscious in the person and represents the reality of the outside world to the self. Psychoanalysis has an eye for unconscious psychological conflicts, especially between personal, bodily desires and social taboos. It also takes seriously emotions, neuroses, sexuality, and mental illness. Psychoanalysis in general has made historians much more aware of the unconscious in their subjects' lives instead of automatically assuming the rationality of behaviour, although few historians have worked explicitly with psychoanalytic theory. Historians often object to its universal, timeless, and biological assumptions and its presumed circularity and unfalsifiability.[81]

Exceptionally, the historian Lyndal Roper applies psychoanalytic insights in her work on early modern witchcraft. Lyndal Roper builds on the work of the psychoanalyst Melanie Klein (1882–1960), who was preoccupied with the frustrations a baby experiences in relation to the mother's breast, and the good and bad associations with this breast in the child's phantasy. Lyndal Roper noted a pattern in early modern accusations of witchcraft. The accusers were mothers who had just had a baby, and the accused were lying-in maids: older, child-less women who had assisted in the mothers' households during the first weeks after childbirth. These 'barren' lying-in maids were thought to feel envy towards the family they worked for, and witches were seen as harming people directly by their envy, causing physical hurt by projecting their emotions onto bodies. Roper notes that the signs of witchcraft were found on the babies' bodies, and that the language of the accusation revolved around nourishment, oral satisfac-tion, the breast, and milk:

> The food the witch gave the mother was sprinkled with white or black diabolic powders or the soups she was fed were poisonous; and these of course influenced the milk the infant received in a very immediate way [...] the infant's feeding had been disrupted so that no satisfactory nourishing could take place and the relation between mother and child was destroyed.[82]

Motherhood was the dominant theme in the witch trials. Instead of looking for other causes – such as conflicts over charity, property, or power, or evidence of sexual antagonism between men and women – as other historians have done, Roper focuses on motherhood and its relationship with subjectivity. The main motifs of the accusations were 'suckling, giving birth, food and feeding'.[83] This can be explained by a psychoanalytical emphasis on early childhood. Roper stresses anxiety as part of the period directly after childbirth, both because of high child mortality and the risk that this period will trigger the mother's mem-ories of when she was a baby herself, including feelings of hate and love towards her own mother. If her baby died or fell ill, Roper speculates, these early child-hood memories (and possibly ambivalent feelings towards the newborn baby) could lead to a projection of guilt and anxiety onto the lying-in maid, who was then accused of being a witch: 'The lying-in maid was thus destined for the role of evil mother, because she could be seen to use her feminine power to give oral gratification to do the reverse – to suck the infant dry, poison the mother and her milk [...]'.[84] This mechanism that Klein coined as 'splitting' (projecting intolerable feelings of hostility onto someone else), can, according to Roper, have different expressions in different cultures: modern women may be more likely to internalize feelings of guilt and suffer from post-natal depression. In

this model, psychic conflicts seem to be universal, but their expression is historically variable.

Roper aims to remedy the denial of the body in feminist history by gauging the
'physiological and psychological reality' of gender, as different from a linguistic
cultural construction:

> The body as we experience it is more than the sum of tactile and kinetic impres-
> sions. Our experience of the body is organized by body images. These are in part
> culturally created, and to that extent they have a collective history. We gain
> access to these only partially through language, and it is misleading, I think, to
> equate them with discourse or language. [...] I want to delineate the only par-
> tially conscious images of the body which lie below the surface of language.[85]

Against the accusation that psychoanalysis is ahistorical, Roper holds that it can
help historians to historicize subjectivity, in particular to conceptualize the relation of mind and body and distinguish this from more universal psychic structures such as phantasy, the unconscious, and the centrality of parental figures in
psychic life.[86] In this perspective, gendered subjectivities are both socially and discursively constructed, but also have unchanging, ahistorical, mental elements.[87]
For Roper, a psychoanalytical method is inextricably connected to the history of
the body, since we need to know more about how bodily experiences influence
culture and (sexual) subjectivity, and about the place of the irrational in social
life. The advantage of psychoanalytic approaches is that they address individual
subjectivity, in contrast to the collective concept of subjectivity, which can be
found in the work of Foucault, Weber, and Elias.[88] A psychoanalytical approach
thus highlights emotions, the body, and the unconscious.

▶ Conclusion

This chapter has offered an overview of theories concerned with reconstructing
and explaining the bodily experiences of people in the past. The phenomenological approach of the philosopher Merleau-Ponty rejected Cartesian dualism by
focusing on the body subject. In addition, it stressed the connections between
the individual body and its environment. Although Fanon and Young found
phenomenology's emphasis on lived experience productive, they also criticized

Merleau-Ponty's approach for providing a universal narrative that did not apply to black people or women, respectively. Thus, the phenomenological account of subjective and individual embodiment has been accused of being 'largely devoid of historical and sociological content', of neglecting physical differences, power, and the influence of social structures on bodies.[89]

Historians applying a phenomenological approach have used it to lay bare the lived experience of the body in the past, rather than merely reconstructing discourses or facts. The notion of experience can therefore serve to connect macro- and micro-history.[90] Phenomenology can provide a way to bridge dualisms such as body–mind and inner–outer, but also to link the individual to his or her surroundings. So far, historians and literary scholars have not used phenomenology as a method very often. Bruce Smith suggests this is because phenomenology revolves around relationships, rather than tangible objects; because it seems to be too much about subjective experience and not about objective reconstructions; and because its method is rather loosely described.[91] In addition, historians have struggled with finding primary sources that address emotions and the body, and with the problem of the representation of bodily experience in textual sources.

To explain the reproduction of classed, bodily behaviour in the past, historians have also resorted to Bourdieu's notion of habitus, which emphasizes that corporeal motions are learned and internalized. The concept of habitus was formulated to incorporate cultural and familial norms and hence seems open to historical change. It thus seems less universal than phenomenologists' idea of embodiment. Still, it is argued that both phenomenology and the notion of habitus do not sufficiently discuss inner experience. Therefore psychoanalysis suggests we pay more attention to the unconscious in relation to bodily experience, to 'imaginary bodies'.[92] However, psychoanalytical and phenomenological approaches are not mutually exclusive, as we have seen in Fanon's work. Where phenomenology directs us to the connections between the body and its environment, psychoanalysis may bring us one step further in exploring the individually, interiorly lived body.

6 Materialist Approaches to the Body

▶ Introduction

In the preceding chapters, we have confronted the limitations of several theoretical approaches when it comes to reconstructing historical bodily experience. We have seen how social constructionist approaches have been welcomed for paying attention to cultural variability in representing the body, but have also been criticized for not addressing the material, biological body. Phenomenological approaches, on the other hand, do attempt to reconstruct and analyze bodily experience, but have also proved problematic because of the limitations of primary sources regarding (individual) corporeal experience. In many theories, moreover, individual, bodily agency is found to be lacking. In this final chapter, therefore, I discuss a new branch of theoretical approaches that claims to put the material body at the centre of the analysis. I first discuss approaches that emphasize the biological aspects of the body, and then a diverse set of theories that can be grouped under the heading 'new materialism'. New materialism seeks new theoretical approaches that go beyond discourse analysis.[1] It can be seen as a critique of the late twentieth-century dominance of the linguistic paradigm in the humanities, as well as a re-examination of the central place of the human being, focusing rather on the connections between humans and non-humans such as objects, animals, plants, and the environment. It thus foregrounds 'matter'.

An early symbol of this new materialism is the figure of the cyborg, as presented by the biologist and feminist science scholar Donna Haraway in 1985. In Haraway's vision, the cyborg – a human whose body is augmented by technological parts – personifies both an emerging technoculture characterized by increasingly intimate relationships between the body and machines and 'a creature in a post-gender world'.[2] With this partly fictional figure, Haraway sought to criticize those strands of feminism who associated women with nature and idealized this connection. The cyborg epitomized the breaking down of binary oppositions such as nature–culture, biological–technical, self–other, female–male, and body–mind, all dualisms that had contributed to the domination of women, people of colour, nature, workers, and animals.[3]

Haraway's questioning of dichotomies, especially the one between human and non-human, would become a central feature of new materialist theory. In this chapter I address the theoretical implications of this 'material turn' for conceptualizations of the body, but also the practical ways in which historians can apply new materialist approaches to their studies of the body in the past.

▶ History, biology, and the neurosciences

Before the rise of the 'new cultural history' in the 1980s and 1990s, which was influenced by poststructuralism and centred around representations and discourse, the body had often unproblematically been regarded as a natural, biological element. The cultural turn, on the other hand, underlined the cultural construction of the body. This raised the question of the exact nature of the relationship between nature and culture. In this section a number of scholars are discussed who have argued that historians should take serious account of biology and other natural sciences in writing the history of humanity, bodies, emotions, and disease. These scholars are generally considered 'materialists', and should be distinguished from the 'new materialists', discussed later in this chapter.

For the major part of the twentieth century, historians assumed that the body was ancient, but the mind was young, our large brain only gaining its present form around 4000 BCE when tools came to be used. This assumption is based on a strict Cartesian distinction between an unchanging body and a developing brain. As the historian Daniel Lord Smail argues, not only does the brain have a much longer history, but the noncognitive features of the brain – such as behavioural dispositions and emotions – have a deep evolutionary history. Smail builds on recent work in neuropsychology and neurophysiology that has demonstrated that body states like the emotions are located in specific parts of the brain, and that they owe their location to natural selection. Most of these body states are facilitated or blocked by chemicals such as hormones and neurotransmitters.

Smail proposes a history built on these new insights from neuropsychology and neurophysiology, a 'neurohistorical approach':

> The existence of brain structures and body chemicals means that predisposi-
> tions and behavioural patterns have a biological substrate that simply cannot be
> ignored [...]. The neurohistorical approach embraces the recent interest in cog-
> nition as well as all histories that emphasize noncognitive aspects of the brain,
> including the history of emotions. But to acknowledge the physical or neural
> reality of moods and predispositions is not to adopt a crude genetic determin-
> ism. Even less does it invoke the illusory search for an essential human nature
> engineered by natural selection in the distant past [...].[4]

Smail highlights that behaviours that are shaped by predispositions and emotions are at the same time shaped by different historical cultures. He regards
the body states generated by activities of the brain and the endocrine system
as a backdrop of feelings, which, however, do not dictate behaviour. They
form the preconditions for people's decision making. Thus, Smail clearly dis-
tances himself from a crude biological determinism. Instead, he emphasizes
the interrelationship between biology and culture, between genes and the
environment: 'cultural practices can have profound neurophysiological consequences'.[5]

One example of 'neurohistory' concerns a new regime of 'brain–body chemistry', which surfaced in the last 5,000 years, according to Smail, but accelerated in
the long eighteenth century, the 'century of addiction'.[6] This century witnessed a
significant expansion in a range of mood-altering consumption items like coffee,
tea, sugar, chocolate, and tobacco, new recreational drugs such as nitrous oxide
and opium, but also exciting activities such as the reading of novels and erotic
literature – widely regarded as addictive stimulants of women's passions, especially – and gossiping, facilitated by new sociable venues like cafés and salons.
Smail refers to all these modern mood-altering practices as 'psychotropic mech-
anisms', which together form a 'psychotropic economy'. He suggests that the
new regime of addictive items for consumption replaced religion and rituals as
sources of stimulants, concluding that a neurohistorical approach 'offers a new
interpretative framework, where human neurophysiology is one of the environmental factors in macrohistorical change'.[7] Rather than focusing on new inventions and ideas – often seen as part of civilizational progress by historians – Smail

proposes that we should also consider that this might be explained by nothing more than changing body chemistry.[8]

Although Smail's emphasis on actual bodily effects of new patterns of consumption is important, and certainly makes up for a limited cultural–historical discursive approach to these changes or a socio-economic description of consumption patterns, the historical evidence for these developments remains scant. Other studies by scientists from various disciplines, including feminist science scholars, demonstrate in more detail how biology and culture, or nature and nurture, always interact, for example as the brain adapts to the environment.[9] Biology here becomes much more than a static and essentialist focus on nature. Instead, throughout the life course bodies continually change, their initial biological set-up being influenced by cultural circumstances and vice versa. The question here is how historians can trace this interaction, especially since it is hard to keep up with the fast-changing research in the sciences.[10] For historians the issue of how we might theorize the body as 'simultaneously composed of genes, hormones, cells, and organs – all of which influence health and behaviour – and of culture and history'[11] remains a vexed question, especially since so few primary sources include references to physical change in bodies over time.

▷ New materialism: Karen Barad

Whereas Smail's work is positioned very much in line with the neurosciences, recent more theoretical work in the humanities aims to combine insights from the natural sciences with philosophy and cultural theory. The body is just one theme among many covered by these 'new materialist' approaches, which are largely grounded in feminist theory. One influential poststructuralist feminist theorist who put the notion of matter on the agenda is Judith Butler. As we have seen in Chapter 4, Butler asks how bodies come to matter: 'What are the constraints by which bodies are materialized as "sexed," and how are we to understand the "matter" of sex, and of bodies more generally, as the repeated and violent circumscription of cultural intelligibility? Which bodies come to matter – and why?'[12] Why, Butler wonders, are some bodies seen as abnormal or 'abject', as is the case, for instance, with transgender bodies, which are often regarded as not being 'properly gendered', and thus do not 'matter'? Butler proposes to 'return to the notion of matter, not as site or surface, but as *a process of materialization that stabilizes over time to produce the effect of boundary, fixity, and surface we call matter.'*[13] Although Butler explicitly states that she does not claim that discourse 'originates, causes, or exhaustively composes that which it concedes', her work has nevertheless been interpreted by many readers as solely capturing the discursive construction of (material and sexed) bodies and as reducing materiality to *'merely* an effect of power'.[14] Feminist theorists have therefore sought to expand on Butler's work to think through the material body.

These new materialist approaches often stem from feminist science studies. The physicist Karen Barad, one of the leading theorists of new materialism, questions the primacy of the cultural turn's emphasis on discourse and representation, but at the same time builds on the poststructuralist philosophies of Butler and Foucault by using the notion of a materialist and **posthumanist** performativity. Whereas Butler highlights the socio-political interpellation of the human subject and the (gendered) materialization of bodies, Barad not only broadens the notion of bodies to include non-human bodies, but also pays attention to 'material-discursive practices' that engender the differences between, for example, human and non-human bodies.[15] Barad no longer wants to think in binary oppositions such as nature–culture, human–nonhuman, realism–social constructivism, or subject–object, but assumes that nature shapes culture and vice versa, without pinpointing points of origin. Similarly, Haraway had already coined the notion of 'naturecultures', the idea that 'bodies and meanings coshape one another'.[16]

Barad proposes what she calls an 'agential realist' perspective on the world and knowledge practices. This **agential realism** involves a relational focus on 'intra-actions' between subjects or objects, which are no longer seen as separate but as entangled 'material-discursive' phenomena:

All bodies, not merely 'human' bodies, come to matter through the world's iterative intra-activity – its performativity. This is true not only of the surface or contours of the body but also of the body in the fullness of its physicality, including the very 'atoms' of its being. Bodies are not objects with inherent boundaries and properties; they are material-discursive phenomena. [...] What is at issue is not some ill-defined process by which human-based linguistic practices (materially supported in some unspecified way) manage to produce substantive bodies/bodily substances but rather a material dynamics of intra-activity: material apparatuses produce material phenomena through specific causal intra-actions, where 'material' is always already material-discursive – *that is what it means to matter.*[17]

Barad thus shifts the theoretical focus from questions of correspondence between descriptions and reality to matters of practices, doings, and actions.[18] Without from the start relying on notions such as inside or outside or the human as either cause or effect, her agential realist account 'acknowledge[s] nature, the body, and materiality in the fullness of their becoming'.[19]

Barad can be seen as one of the founders of the theory of 'new materialism'. Key points made by new materialists include firstly a criticism of binaries such as nature-culture or subject-object. Secondly, new materialism is a new way of doing theory. New materialist scholars do not reject earlier theoretical paradigms, but rather aim to read new theorists in conversation with earlier paradigms as well as with ideas stemming from the natural sciences.[20] Thirdly, and perhaps most importantly, in these approaches matter takes a central position.

One example of historical work on the body that has used Barad's new material-ist approach is Anu Salmela's analysis of female suicides in late nineteenth-century Finland. Drawing on Barad's notion of agential realism, Salmela questions whether suicide was a thoroughly human phenomenon and instead includes the agency of the dead body in her historical narration. The author argues that the nature of female suicide was shaped during autopsies, which, following Barad, can be regarded as 'intra-actions', or encounters between bodies, doctors, and medical dis-course. Bodies and doctors only emerged as separate agents through the post-mor-tem: 'Thus the autopsies were, to use Barad's term, *apparatuses*, socio-material practices that drew boundaries between bodies and doctors.'[21] The autopsy as appa-ratus is the practice in which suicide is shaped. Since the determination of suicide depended on the condition of the body, especially with regard to pronouncements on the mental state of the deceased (often the condition of the uterus was seen to be related to the mind), Salmela concludes that the body participated actively in giving meaning to the mental state, and hence also to the manner of burial, which depended on whether or not the suicide was intentional. Decayed cadavers could, moreover, prevent the dissection and thus the autopsy. She thus states that death was 'a doing' and that matter had agency.[22] In addition, Salmela concludes that agential realism 'provides a non-deterministic framework for exploring the past'.[23] Instead of focusing on the end results, which have already defined an object as such, agential realism may help us notice the formative moment of historical phenomena, not initially assuming that objects have a certain form. A focus on the role of matter, Salmela proposes, can help the historian see that 'a historical happening is a material-discursive becoming, an on-going and intra-active mate-rialization of the world'[24]: since the bodies of suicides differed, the determination of suicide in the apparatus of the post-mortem did too.

The new materialist allocation of agency to material objects, in this case the dead body, has caused some upheaval among historians and other scholars. They retort that human agency is of a different quality than that of matter. Barad herself has remarked on agency being asymmetrical, since it is humans who are in the position to represent the world,[25] as is pointed out by Salmela. Whether these dead bodies had a similar type of agency to that of doctors is questionable, then, but Salmela's emphasis on the role of matter in the autopsy is innovative: instead of merely reconstructing the medical discourse, historians can now also include the dead body as agent and part of an apparatus in their accounts. Barad's insights for historians imply a focus not only on agential matter, but also on intra-actions or socio-material practices, in which the material and discursive are entwined. Last, this type of new materialist analysis may provide a more open framework for studying the origins of historical formations, instead of their outcomes.

▶ New materialism: Gilles Deleuze and the 'becoming' body

The notion of **potentiality** is also strongly linked with the philosophy of Gilles Deleuze (1925–1995), which inspired another theoretical strand of new materialism. Although some philosophers question the extent to which Deleuze's body of thought can be classified as new materialism,[26] his philosophy has been important to those scholars searching for the foundations of that approach. Deleuze, in turn, was strongly influenced by the work of the seventeenth-century Dutch Jewish philosopher Baruch Spinoza (1632–1677). Spinoza asked the question: What can a body do? In formulating this question, Spinoza rejected the Cartesian mind-body dualism and its accompanying hierarchy and replaced it with 'parallelism', implying that body and mind must be conceived in parallel: we can come to know our body via our mind and vice versa, since what affects our mind simultaneously affects our body.[27] In this view, the body should be seen neither as an object or a given nor as a vehicle of the mind. As Deleuze and his co-author Félix Guattari put it:

> We know nothing about a body until we know what it can do, in other words, what its affects are, how they can or cannot enter into composition with other affects, with the affects of another body, either to destroy that body or to be destroyed by it, either to exchange actions and passions with it or to join with it in composing a more powerful body.[28]

Deleuze and Guattari emphasize the potential of the body or, in a Deleuzian phrase, its 'becoming'. As Ian Buchanan notes, 'By making the question of what a body can do constitutive, what Deleuze and Guattari effectively do is reconfigure the body as the sum of its capacities'.[29] A Deleuzian analysis of the body thus focuses on affects and relations, where affect can be seen as the capacity of a body to form specific relations, that is, the virtual links between bodies.[30] Health in this line of thinking means the actual measurable capacity to form new relations. Healthy relations are those which ensure the formation of new compounds. For example, the ability to gather food and eat it might seem exterior to the body, but is in fact vital to any definition of the body: 'Health, then, is the happy union of a capacity to form new relations and the new relations themselves, which in their turn permit the body to go on to form other new relations.'[31]

Relations, becoming, and potential are key words in Deleuze's vocabulary. Deleuze argues against the idea, promulgated by Freud's psychoanalysis, for example, that individuals are driven by involuntary instincts, since this focus may obscure relations. As Scott Lash points out: 'For Deleuze, the body is the surface of intersection between libidinal forces, on the one hand, and "external", social forces on the other.'[32] Deleuze's focus on relationships is also central in the notion of 'assemblage' or 'machine', which dismisses the view that the relationships of component parts are stable and fixed; rather these heterogeneous composites can shift and reshift within and among other bodies, initiating alignments with other bodies, objects, or ideas, and responding to those items. Deleuze and Guattari therefore speak of a 'body without organs' to highlight that we should not experience our bodies in terms of biology. Instead, the body without organs is a body full of potential, a body that increases the number of ways it can affect and be affected by other bodies.[33] The body here can refer to human, animal, textual, social, cultural, and physical bodies; it is denaturalized and yet at the same time not fixed by structures or regulations.[34]

Appetite, for instance, is often conceived as a bodily drive, in which the free mind is obscured by bodily needs. For Deleuze, however, appetite and the body need to be placed in relation to food and the affections deriving from it.[35] Deleuze observes this process in his analysis of anorexia. He critiques a psychoanalytical or psychiatric pre-established explanation of anorexia that presumes it is a disorder caused by unsuccessfully repressed past trauma. Instead Deleuze problematizes the notion of 'disorder', and rather than searching for origins, highlights the ongoing acts of the anorexic:

> The anorexic consists of a body without organs with voids and fulnesses. [...] It is not a matter of a refusal of the body, it is a matter of the refusal of the organism, of a refusal of what the organism makes the body undergo. Not regression at all, but involution, involuted body. The anorexic void has nothing to do with a lack, it is on the contrary a way of escaping the organic constraint of lack and hunger at the mechanical mealtime. [...] Anorexia is a political system, a micro-politics: to escape from the norms of consumption in order not to be an object of consumption oneself. It is a feminine protest, from a woman who wants to have a functioning of the body and not simply organic and social functions which make her dependent. [...] In short, anorexia is a history of politics: to be the involuted of the organism, the family or the consumer society. There is politics as soon as there is a continuum of intensities (anorexic food and fullness), emission and conquest of food particles (constitution of a body without organs, in opposition to a dietary or organic regime), and above all combination of fluxes (the food flux enters into relation with a clothes flux, a flux of language, a flux of sexuality: a whole, molecular woman-becoming in the anorexic [...]).[36]

Deleuze here maps what is going on with the anorexic, who is always in a dynamic relation to many other elements (food, family, ideology of consumption). Rather than interpreting anorexia as a lack of appetite, Deleuze assumes it is built on a female desire: anorexia is not a refusal of the body, but a refusal of a certain ideology of the body. This ideology includes notions of 'proper' femininity and 'proper' eating at mealtimes. The anorexic, however, 'betrays' natural hunger as well as the family that insists on a common meal. Experimenting with 'void' and 'fullness', for instance by picking up morsels of food, the anorexic is the process of becoming woman.[37]

Deleuze saw a correspondence between his notion of the body and Merleau-Ponty's phenomenological 'lived body', except that he refused to attribute the 'unity, coherence and intentionality to the body' that can be found in Merleau-Ponty's view of the body.[38] Similarly to Merleau-Ponty's, the Deleuzian framework attempts to transcend binaries, including those between the real and representation. The social, exterior and the psychical, interior are not opposites, but are intermingled.[39] Perhaps what makes Deleuze's work on the body stand out most is his emphasis on 'becoming'. Nevertheless, Deleuze's ideas on the body remain open to discussion.[40]

Few historians so far have applied Deleuze's approaches to the history of the body. One exception is the historian Lisa Helps. Helps finds Deleuze's ideas on the body helpful since they regard the body as desiring to connect with other organic and inorganic bodies to form assemblages, particular configurations of living beings and things, which come together at particular times and places. This emphasis on assemblages highlights the dynamic aspects of bodies as becoming. Helps takes as an example the historical case study of Joseph J., a man brought before the police court in Victoria, British Columbia in 1881 after he had fled to Washington but returned on the next steamer. He was sentenced to three months' hard labour breaking rocks in the chain gang for loitering in the street and vagrancy. Whereas a Foucauldian approach would interpret this judicial procedure as one of discipline and normalization of the convict's body, Helps proposes a Deleuzian take:

> We might also think of Joseph J. as a 'boat-man-water assemblage', however, deterritorializing, fleeing to Washington, and becoming, through desire (desire to return to Victoria, desire to loiter and smoke with his friends, desire to be affected by tobacco and conversation in a familiar place), a road-man-tobacco assemblage. By arresting Joseph J., the superintendent of police (a gun-man-tobacco assemblage) blocked this desiring assemblage, he reterritorialized it, removed it from the street, and impeded it from embodying public space in seemingly undesirable ways. The magistrate coded the road-man-tobacco assemblage as 'vagrant' and again reterritorialized this assemblage through hard labour in the prison to becoming a chain-man-rock assemblage. In these two different readings, I am not merely saying the same thing in different words; in the disciplinary and normalizing reading of the body, systems of power, and, of course, resistance to these systems – perhaps Joseph J. refused to work – make the body. In the second reading, it is desire that drives becoming and systems of power that bind or block this becoming.[41]

Helps builds on the Deleuzian take on the body's capacity to affect and be affected to argue that it is the power of the body to connect that is important here, rather than the power imposed on the body by the penal system. Thus, Helps proposes that historians historically scrutinize the making and unmaking of the assemblages the body forms, rather than assuming that the body is a stable unit of analysis. In addition, if we accept the primary assumption of the body as desiring to connect with other bodies, then we might interpret systems of power such as the penal system as reactive, as trying to hold back the desiring bodies. From this perspective, Helps suggests, the body might be seen as the motor of history.[42]

A Deleuzian reading, therefore, is an *affirmative* reading of the potentiality of the body.[43] This reading of the body as full of active desire is often opposed to Foucault's notion of the disciplined body, an object to reactive normalizing and individuating forces.[44] On the other hand, Deleuze's views on the body are also contrasted with the importance attached by phenomenology to intentionality and to the psychoanalytical view of the body as a mode of expression of inner feelings.[45] As Elizabeth Grosz formulates it:

> The body is thus not an organic totality which is capable of the wholesale expression of subjectivity, a welling up of the subject's emotions, attitudes, beliefs, or experiences, but is itself an assemblage of organs, processes, pleasures, passions, activities, behaviors linked by fine lines and unpredictable networks to other elements, segments, and assemblages.[46]

In short, Deleuze proposes seeing the potential of the body, and its desire to form relationships with other bodies. Like other new materialist theorists, Deleuze rejects binaries such as body–mind or real–representation, but attempts to combine all these factors in the notion of dynamic assemblages. Deleuze's work has been central to the so-called non-human turn, the recent critical reappraisal of the privilege given to the human in a world consisting of so many other entities such as animals, objects, plants, and the environment.[47]

▷ Science and technology studies and the body: Bruno Latour

Another strand of new materialism, which describes matter in a more practical and, to a certain extent, less theoretical way, is Science and Technology Studies (STS). STS scholars study science in practice or, in the words of one of its foremost proponents, the French philosopher, anthropologist, and sociologist Bruno Latour (1947–), 'science in action'. In his book *The Pasteurization of France* (1988) Latour traces the history of microbes by focusing not on the genius of one scientist, Louis Pasteur, but on the 'networks' consisting of scientists, laboratories, instruments, bureaucrats, and organic matter. Instead of presenting one human scientist as discovering an inert passive element of nature, Latour gives agency to matter (the microbes), thereby deconstructing the human–nonhuman binary and expanding the agentic factors into a network of multiple forces both social, economic, and political. His focus on networks also surfaced in his Actor-Network Theory (ANT).[48]

Applied to the body, Latour's insights imply that we dismiss the subject–object model, in which a subjective, experiencing body is opposed to a natural world consisting of objects. For Latour, what is missing in this model is the 'learning of the body to be affected': Rather than defining the body as a (natural) essence, Latour proposes that the body be regarded as

> *an interface that becomes more and more describable as it learns to be affected by more and more elements.* The body is thus not a provisional residence of something superior – an immortal soul, the universal or thought – but what leaves a dynamic trajectory by which we learn to register and become sensitive to what the world is made of. [...] there is no sense in defining the body directly, but only in rendering the body sensitive to what these other elements are.[49]

Latour gives the example of the training of 'noses' for the perfume industry through the use of odour kits consisting of a series of distinct pure fragrances. These contrasts between the different odours need to be learned in a training session, which ends successfully when the trainee can discriminate ever more subtle differences in fragrance and is able to distinguish them from one another. The trainee is then called 'a nose', since it seems that only this practice has given her this body organ: 'she learned to have a nose that allowed her to inhabit a (richly differentiated odoriferous) world. Thus body parts are progressively acquired at the same time as "world counter-parts" are being registered in a new way. Acquiring a body is thus a progressive enterprise that produces at once a sensory medium *and* a sensitive world.'[50] Latour sees the odour kit as a part of the body as understood as 'training to be affected'. The kit functions as coextensive with the body because it trains the nostrils and makes odours that affect the trained 'nose' who engages in smelling.[51] In short, Latour incorporates objects into body practices and has an eye for the dynamic learning of the body. Networks in which the body is connected with objects and the environment are central in his work, and in this way Latour attempts to go beyond dualistic concepts such as nature–nurture. This endeavour to transcend dualisms runs through all kinds of new materialist approaches.

▶ Praxiography: Annemarie Mol and Amade M'Charek

Building on insights from STS, a number of scholars have coined the methodology of 'praxiography'. In this section, I first discuss how praxiography has been applied by anthropologists and sociologists, and then how historians have worked with this approach.

Annemarie Mol (1958–), an ethnographer, empirical philosopher and medical doctor, proposed applying a praxiographical approach to the body, in particular to the disease of atherosclerosis, a hardening of the arteries. As an ethnographer doing fieldwork, Mol observed patients with atherosclerosis in a Dutch hospital. The results of her observations were published in *The Body Multiple: Ontology in Medical Practice* (2002). Mol notes that the disease atherosclerosis differs according to the medical practice or technology: this disease can be identified in tissue of corpses studied under a microscope, through X-rays, or through a conversation in which a patient explains what he or she is feeling. Mol then argues that different techniques produce different bodies, hence *the body multiple*. Crucially, for Mol this is not a repetition of the idea that the body is culturally constructed, which would imply that there is one (natural) body, and several perspectives on that body, for example the doctor's and the patient's. This **perspectivalism** foregrounds meanings and interpretations of the body, but neglects the body's physical reality or the disease itself. Moreover, Mol argues that this perspectivalism leaves the physical body untouched, whereas she aims to bring the disease itself back into view.[52]

So instead of perspectivalism, Mol focuses on ontology, which is shaped in daily practices, claiming that diseases are *enacted*, that is, done in practices with the help of different techniques.[53] The term enactment has been chosen carefully, to indicate more flexibility than the term 'construction', and to pay more attention to the shifting ontologies, whose identities may differ between sites.[54] Mol, like Latour, attempts to go beyond dualisms such as object–subject or doctor–patient:

> This, then, may be a way out of the dichotomy between the knowing subject and the objects-that-are-known: to spread the activity of knowing widely. To spread it out over tables, knives, records, microscopes, buildings, and other things or habits in which it is embedded. Instead of talking about subjects *knowing* objects we may then, as a next step, come to talk about *enacting* reality in practice.[55]

Mol's focus on practices in which a disease is enacted also highlights which actions take place in order to warrant coherence: for instance, to ensure that one can continue to speak of 'the' disease of atherosclerosis, as happens in a hospital. The patient file is one of those means of creating coherence. There, all the different techniques used to examine the patient come together under the label 'atherosclerosis'. The body, in short, may be multiple, but practices of coordination can help us navigate this multiplicity.[56]

Mol's praxiography thus dismisses binary categories and focuses on the enactment of the body in various practices, with an eye for techniques, instruments, and objects, like Latour's ANT. What this approach seems to lack is an attention to cultural context and a political critique, which were prominent in social constructionist theories of the body presented by, for example, Laqueur or Butler.

Several other scholars have applied praxiography to topics relating to the body. One example is the work by the anthropologist Amade M'Charek on race, which shows how race is enacted in different practices. One practice M'Charek studies is the role of CCTV in identifying suspects. In 2006 a 17-year-old boy was murdered in the main hall of Brussels Railway Station. CCTV footage showed the victim being stabbed by two boys of the same age. The police released the CCTV video to the media and asked the public to help identify the suspects, whom they thought to be of North African, probably Moroccan, descent. In the media the suspects' clothing (Nike sneakers and sweatshirts) and body movement played a large role. Their behaviour of hanging around the station was regarded as suspect. M'Charek observes that in this case Moroccan-ness was not simply established on the basis of externally visible traits, but rather 'was based on a series of links established between location, clothing, and appearance as well as the framing of this all through the invested technology of CCTV, a technology that is, as it were, criminalized and often racialized.'[57] More generally, she finds that race can be enacted as colour, national descent, clothing, body movements, location, narrative, DNA, and physical appearance. M'Charek therefore concludes that 'race cannot be reduced to one marker of difference'.[58]

Thus M'Charek argues that race is enacted in relations, as well as being material and multiple. She explicitly aims to go beyond the binary distinction between the biological and the social by arguing that race is a relational object. Following Mol, M'Charek contends that race is multiple: 'The difference between multiple and plural is crucial. To say that different relational configurations make *different versions of race* is radically different from saying that race might assume *different meanings* in different contexts.'[59] In short, M'Charek highlights the materiality of race, without fixing or naturalizing it. She is inspired by STS to look at configurations (of race), including material practices and technologies. Like Mol, she studies the ontology of bodies, underlining their multiplicity and relationality.

▶ Praxiography and history: Geertje Mak

In this section, I examine how historians have applied ideas from praxiography. The example comes from the history of intersex people (in the past referred to as hermaphrodites), who were born with ambiguous sexual characteristics. Historians have argued that the era of modern medicalization led to the enforcement of a sex by physicians onto their intersex patients. Alice Dreger, for instance, identifies a shift to the 'age of gonads' (1870–1915): at this time, physicians and scientists, when faced with cases of 'doubtful sex', decided, in order to uphold the strict separation between male and female or sexual dimorphism, that only gonadal tissue – the presence of either ovarian or testicular tissue – determined 'true sex'. Regardless of other physical or mental characteristics, the presence of either gonadal issue would immediately lead to the classification of the individual as a man or a woman.[60] However, historian Geertje Mak argues that this medicalization was not complete, and she uses a praxiographic approach to make this argument. Studying mostly medical sources, in which doctors sometimes meticulously noted the techniques they used to examine the body and establish sex, Mak concludes that from the first decade of the twentieth century, sex was determined not only by the gonads, but also by the 'self' of the hermaphrodite. Whereas in the early modern period most hermaphrodites were accepted by the local community as long as they were not sexually active, from 1870 'sex' shifted from a moral position to a corporeal meaning. Sex came to depend on the functioning of the body, especially with regard to menstruation and sexual intercourse. And when, from the late nineteenth century, the increasing number of operations led to more cases of hermaphrodites being discovered by accident, this paved the way for adding the 'self' as a major criterion for classifying the hermaphrodite as man or woman. So although in the modern period the treatment of hermaphrodites was problematized and medicalized, doctors were not all-powerful: they took into account their patients' own sense of sexual identity.[61]

As a case study, Mak presents the case of Louise-Julia-Anna from 1893. She was raised as a girl and visited a doctor because of complaints relating to what later turned out to be a hernia in the groin area. The French physician François Guermonprez, based in Lille, was requested to examine Louise-Julia-Anna. He looked at the hernia and palpated and touched it to establish whether it was a testicle, but this was not self-evident. As Mak states, 'the one and only signifier of sex itself appears in multiple manifestations – seen and measured from the outside, percussed and listened to, touched and felt, laid bare and seen, extracted and microscopically examined.'[62] Furthermore, Guermonprez inspected his patient in different poses, both naked and in a dress, and described her appearance, attitude towards him, emotional reactions, life history, family circumstances, and sexual behaviour. Mak therefore concludes that the *'whole body and person'* was used as evidence to confirm the masculinity that the testicle was invoked to prove: 'In practice, therefore, there is no final physical signifier of sex – signifiers of masculinity continue to refer to *each other*, never to a final "truth".'[63]

By following Mol's focus on medical practices and techniques, Mak aims to demonstrate how sex is *enacted* in the clinical encounter. Like Mol and other new materialists, Mak wants to go beyond the binary opposition between a medically defined, objective sex and the subjective truth of the patient's inner sexed self; instead she aims to question both critically.[64] She argues that different medical practices produce multiple sexes as well as multiple sexed subjectivities. Her praxiographical approach demonstrates that a sole focus on a powerful medical discourse would be insufficient: taking into account practices of examining the body shows us the many forms sex could have in the late nineteenth century. Mak thus also adds a historical framework to her praxiographical approach, which was missing in the work by Mol. Mak builds on Butler's work by taking on Butler's ideas on the discursive and performative construction of gender, yet she also finds this perspective insufficient, since it does not show how gender comes into being *in practice* (and, thus, beyond discourse).

▶ Conclusion

This chapter has considered a number of new materialist approaches to the body. New materialism in general is a relatively recent field of thought that includes a number of diverse strands. The more theoretical strand, including theorists such as Deleuze, Barad, and other feminist philosophers, aims to go beyond the linguistic turn and think through how matter and the body come into being in socio-discursive constellations. These theorists emphasize the need to go beyond binaries such as nature–culture or body–mind, and advocate affirmative readings that promote the becoming of bodies and assemblages.

The more practical strand, deriving from STS and Latour, and including Mol and M'Charek among others, focuses on the practices in which health, the body, race, or gender are enacted. However, these scholars also make theoretical claims deriving from their praxiographic analyses. They want to return to ontology, as evident from the phrase 'the body multiple', and reject binary thinking. Mostly, they are interested in networks and entanglements, in which humans are connected to objects, animals, or other non-human actors.

Historians have, so far, hardly applied the insights from new materialism. I have discussed examples of the few historians who have worked with praxiography, like Mak's praxiographic approach to gender history, Salmela's use of Barad's notion of intra-actions in her socio-material analysis of autopsies in nineteenth-century Finland, and Helps' application of Deleuze's concept of assemblages and his focus on the becoming potential of the body, in contrast to Foucault's underlining of powerful systems that only restrain and discipline bodies. These examples of historical work are innovative and point to the possibilities that new materialism offers historians. However, historians will struggle with the lack of agency found in some new materialist theory, especially with its critique on anthropocentrism. On the one hand, the focus on the non-human opens up a world that includes animals, objects, and the environment; on the other hand, however, this focus might neglect human and bodily agency. Ultimately, the experiencing, feeling body that we encountered in phenomenological approaches has not yet found a place in new materialist theory.[65]

Lastly, especially compared to the explicit political commentary that was such a prominent feature of poststructuralist analyses, new materialism seems to lack this critical intervention. This apparent absence is increasingly remedied by scholars such as Latour and Mol, who are keen to show how their academic work can contribute to current societal issues such as the care for the environment or globalization.[66] So far, however, in regard to the body this political critique has been less prominent in new materialist work.

Conclusion

Undoubtedly, the rise of body history from the late 1980s was strongly connected to the cultural and linguistic turns. The cultural turn paved the way for an attention to human behaviour in daily life, including illness, health, and sexuality, while the linguistic turn stimulated historians to study representations of gender and the body in symbolic practices, images, and discourses. The latter shift to the representation of the body led to a wealth of studies on the historical framing of diseases such as tuberculosis, hysteria, and anorexia, but also on the construction of gendered bodies and individual body parts, such as the skin or the vagina.[1] These studies have revealed the body as so much more than a natural, biological entity and have given us insight into the historically variable meanings projected onto bodies. They have demonstrated how the body is often used (or abused) by political ideology, how difference is attached to bodies, but also how the body is made productive, especially in the modern era.[2] In short, the history of the body has been a fruitful lens through which to approach not only social and cultural history, but also history writing more broadly. As Roger Cooter notes, the 'somatic turn', which was strongly connected with the postmodern linguistic turn, discussed more than just the body as a discrete object of enquiry: 'The "somatic turn" (of which body history was a part) was broadly a means to explicate and illustrate how concepts and categories like "the body" and practices like "history" served to naturalize, rationalize and cohere a reality that was increasingly felt by many late twentieth century intellectuals to be fragmented.'[3] Cooter argues that the corporeal turn problematized an essentialist view of the body, just as it critiqued the modernist notion of objective, coherent history writing.

Evaluating body history as a field more generally, we may conclude that attempts to examine the corporeal in the past have also encountered problems. The focus on the discursive representation of the body, especially, has failed to help us understand individual or collective bodies as feeling, experiencing entities, even though the power of the constructionist perspective lay in presenting historically variable cultural ideas of the body, as well as the ideologies informing those ideas. Similarly, historians have often found that constructionist theories exclude individual agency and the material aspects of the body.

A second problem in body history has been the enduring persistence of Cartesian dualism. The predominance of mind over body has long been regarded as the explanation for the neglect of the body in history and philosophy, a neglect that was remedied by the somatic turn. However, much work in both body history and in cultural theory remained entrenched in the dualism of body and mind, as is evidenced by the recent materialist turn strongly arguing against such dualism and instead advocating a broader perspective based on networks or constellations. We might wonder, though, whether emphatically dismissing body–mind dualism may not further perpetuate this dichotomy by keeping it as a yardstick.

A third problem in body history concerns the boundlessness of the topic of the body, which might reduce its utility for research. This potential criticism can be roundly rebutted by pointing to the wealth of powerful and interesting work that the concept of the body has inspired. Besides, perhaps it is precisely the position of the body at the crossroads of the individual, subjective experience and collective norms that makes it so important for the dynamics of culture.[4] Nevertheless, it is true that the field of the body has expanded enormously, and overlaps with many other fields such as medical history, queer history, gender history, or the history of emotion. The future will tell whether the label of the body will remain the most useful for historians, or whether fields such as the history of the senses, queer history, disability history, or the history of experience will become more dominant.

This book has presented several theoretical perspectives on the body, varying from its cultural construction in discourse, as studied mostly by postmodernist historians, to the ways it moves in and makes sense of the world, as highlighted by phenomenology, and the networks and practices of which the material body is part, as underlined by new materialist scholars. Each body of theory highlights certain aspects of the body, inevitably to the detriment of others. Whereas discursive constructionist approaches have been accused of neglecting individual agency and the material body, new materialist scholars – who have tried to remedy the lack of attention for the material sides of the body and its connections with the environment, other humans, and objects – have thus far had limited success in incorporating the political criticism that was so strong in social constructionist approaches.

One of the solutions might simply be a more eclectic approach: combining a discursive constructionist approach, which deconstructs claims relating to the biological body and demonstrates how the body is ideologically constructed, with a phenomenological take, which studies how individuals experience their bodies in a world which is shaped by ideologies and cultural norms. Postmodern and phenomenological approaches are, in fact, by no means incompatible.[5] I would argue that the notion of embodiment, or the lived body in relation to cultural norms, the environment, and other people, promises the best solution here and has not been explored or applied sufficiently by historians, possibly because they are dependent on the availability of appropriate primary sources. On the basis of these sources it is often easier to deconstruct discourse on the body than to reconstruct individual corporeal experience. The latter aspect is also neglected by new materialism, which, even though it includes material practices in which bodies form part of more elaborate networks, often fails to include a thinking, feeling, experiencing body.

In addition to taking the notion of embodiment more seriously, historians should not forget that the powerful impact of body history derived precisely from its political criticism, laying bare that cultural representations of the body were often purportedly biological, but in fact ideological, if not racist, sexist, or ablist. A critical approach need not be restricted to deconstructing representations of the body; it can also derive from paying more attention to the researcher's reflexivity and emotions during the research process. Some powerful work in the history and sociology of the body has been done by researchers who started from their own bodily experiences, such as black women's encounters with hair,[6] or the experiences of authors suffering from cancer.[7]

Including the historian's body, mind, and emotion as part of the research, and using this to formulate a critical view, can bring back the original power of body history, when it was closely connected with emancipatory movements and the idea of what it meant to be human in the past. This does not mean, however, that the body should be reduced to an entity that is discriminated against. Bodies also display the capacity to experience joy and pleasure. Here, Deleuze's emphasis on the potential of the body to form connections with other bodies might be applied. Moreover, historians who are keen to contextualize bodies in space and time may view the body more dynamically: as Crozier argues, the same body can differ according to locale: 'The body is not used the same way when it is sick, during sex, as it ages, for pleasure, for work, for sport, or when it is represented'. Crozier encourages historians to appreciate this 'underdetermined character' of the body.[8] My hope is that the present overview of historical and theoretical work on the body will inspire historians and future historians to explore these and other uncharted aspects of the human body in history.

Notes

▶ Introduction

1 Jacques Le Goff and Nicolas Truong, *Une Histoire du Corps au Moyen Âge* (Paris, [1983] 2012), p. 1. My translation.

2 Peter Burke, 'Overture: The New History, its Past and its Future', in Peter Burke, ed., *New Perspectives on Historical Writing* (Cambridge, 1991), pp. 2–6.

3 Roy Porter, 'History of the Body', in Peter Burke, ed., *New Perspectives on Historical Writing* (Cambridge, 1991), pp. 206–208.

4 Victoria E. Bonnell and Lynn Hunt, 'Introduction', in Victoria E. Bonnell and Lynn Hunt, eds, *Beyond the Cultural Turn* (Berkeley, CA, 1999), pp. 1–9.

5 Roy Porter, 'History of the Body Reconsidered', in Peter Burke, ed., *New Perspectives on Historical Writing*, 2nd edn (Cambridge, 2001), p. 236.

6 Ibid., p. 253.

7 Ibid., p. 237.

8 Ibid., p. 236.

9 Linda Kalof and William Bynum, eds, *A Cultural History of the Body*, 6 parts (Oxford, 2010); Sarah Toulalan and Kate Fischer, eds, *The Routledge History of Sex and the Body. 1500 to the Present* (London, 2013); Michel Feher, ed., *Fragments for a History of the Human Body*, 3 parts (New York, 1989); Georges Vigarello, ed., *Histoire du Corps*, 3 parts (Paris, 2005).

10 Fay Bound Alberti, *This Mortal Coil. The Human Body in History and Culture* (Oxford, 2016).

11 Bryan S. Turner, *The Body and Society: Explorations in Social Theory*, 3rd edn (London, [1984] 2008); Chris Shilling, *The Body & Social Theory*, 3rd edn (Los Angeles, [1993] 2012); Alexandra Howson, *The Body in Society. An Introduction*, 2nd edn (Cambridge, [2004] 2013); Bryan S. Turner, ed., *Routledge Handbook of Body Studies* (London, 2013). An exception is this introduction to body history in German: Maren Lorenz, *Leibhaftige Vergangenheit. Einführung in die Körpergeschichte* (Tübingen, 2000).

12 Antoinette Burton, 'The Body in/as World History', in Douglas Northrop, ed., *A Companion to World History* (Chichester, 2012), pp. 272–284.

13 Ann-Sophie Lehmann and Herman Roodenburg, eds, *Body and Embodiment in Netherlandish Art. Netherlands Yearbook for the History of Art, 58 (2007–2008)* (Zwolle, 2008); Hans Belting, *An Anthropology of Images. Picture, Medium, Body*, translated by Thomas Dunlap (Princeton, [2011] 2014).

▶ 1   Body, Mind, and Self: Historical Perspectives

1 Daniel H. Garrison, 'Introduction', in Idem, ed., *A Cultural History of the Human Body* (Oxford, 2010), Part 1, 'In Antiquity', p. 7.

2 Patrick Macfarlane, 'Health and Disease', in Garrison, *A Cultural History of the Human Body*, Part 1, 'In Antiquity', p. 46.

3 Anke Bernau, 'Bodies and the Supernatural. Humans, Demons and Angels', in Linda Kalof, ed., *A Cultural History of the Human Body* (Oxford, 2010), Part 2, 'In the Medieval Age', p. 99.

4 Monica H. Green, 'Introduction', in Kalof, ed., *A Cultural History of the Human Body*, Part 2, 'In the Medieval Age', pp. 5–6.

5 Katharine Park, *Secrets of Women: Gender, Generation, and the Origins of Human Dissection* (New York, 2006).

6 Peter Brown, *The Body and Society. Men, Women, and Sexual Renunciation in Early Christianity* (New York, [1988] 2008).

7 Anke Bernau, *Virgins. A Cultural History* (London, 2007), pp. 31–33.

8 Samantha Riches and Bettina Bildhauer, 'Cultural Representations of the Body', in Kalof, ed., *A Cultural History of the Human Body*, Part 2, 'In the Medieval Age', p. 182.

9 Green, 'Introduction', p. 10.

10 Riches and Bildhauer, 'Cultural Representations of the Body', p. 182.

11 Katharine Park, 'Birth and Death', in Kalof, ed., *A Cultural History of the Human Body*, Part 2, 'In the Medieval Age', pp. 33–34.

12 Caroline Bynum, 'Why all the Fuss about the Body? A Medievalist's Perspective', *Critical Inquiry*, 22:1 (1995), p. 13.

13 Caroline Walker Bynum, *The Resurrection of the Body in Western Christianity, 200–1336* (New York, 1995), p. 11.

14 Marie Boas Hall, *The Scientific Renaissance, 1450–1630* (New York, [1962] 1994), p. 129.

15 Roy Porter and Georges Vigarello, 'Corps, Santé et Maladies', in Georges Vigarello, ed., *Histoire du Corps* (Paris, 2005), part I 'De la Renaissance aux Lumières', pp. 361–368.

16 Dalia Judovitz, *The Culture of the Body. Genealogies of Modernity* (Ann Arbor, 2001), pp. 4–5.

17 Jonathan Sawday, *The Body Emblazoned: Dissection and the Human Body in Renaissance Culture* (London, 1995), p. 29.

18 Ibid., p. 265.

19 Mary E. Fissell, *Vernacular Bodies. The Politics of Reproduction in Early Modern England* (Oxford, [2004] 2006).

20 Laura Gowing, *Common Bodies. Women, Touch and Power in Seventeenth-Century England* (New Haven, 2003), pp. 2–6.

21 Ibid., pp. 43–45.

22 Ibid., p. 50.

23 Diane Purkiss, 'The Marked Body: The Witches, Lady Macbeth, and the Relics', in Linda Kalof and William Bynum, eds, *A Cultural History of the Human Body*, Part 3, 'In the Renaissance' (Oxford, 2010), pp. 199–204.

24 Monica H. Green, 'The Diversity of Human Kind', in Kalof, ed., *A Cultural History of the Human Body*, Part 2, 'In the Medieval Age', pp. 173–174.

25 Tony Ballantyne and Antoinette Burton, 'Introduction: Bodies, Empires and World', in Idem, eds, *Bodies in Contact. Rethinking Colonial Encounters in World History* (Durham, 2005), p. 6.

26 Jennifer L. Morgan, 'Male Travelers, Female Bodies, and the Gendering of Racial Ideology, 1500–1770', in Ballantyne and Burton, eds, *Bodies in Contact*, pp. 54–66.

27 Susan Dwyer Amussen, *Caribbean Exchanges: Slavery and the Transformation of English Society, 1640–1700* (Chapel Hill, 2007), p. 134.

28 Londa Schiebinger, 'The Anatomy of Difference: Race and Sex in Eighteenth-Century Science', *Eighteenth-Century Studies*, 23:4 (1990), pp. 392–393.

29 Devin J. Vartija, *The Colour of Equality. Racial Classification and Natural Equality in Enlightenment Encyclopedias* (PhD thesis, Utrecht University, 2018), pp. 26–30.

30 Leonore Davidoff, 'Class and Gender in Victorian England. The Diaries of Arthur J. Munby and Hannah Cullwick', *Feminist Studies*, 5:1 (1979), p. 111.

31 Michael Stolberg, 'Der gesunde Leib. Zur Geschichtlichkeit frühneuzeitlicher Körpererfahrung', in Paul Münch, ed., *'Erfahrung' als Kategorie der Frühneuzeitgeschichte* (Munich, 2001), p. 53.

32 Roy Porter, *Blood and Guts. A Short History of Medicine* (London, [2002] 2003), pp. 75–90.

33 Philipp Sarasin, *Reizbare Maschinen. Eine Geschichte des Körpers 1765–1914* (Frankfurt am Main, 2001), pp. 17–18.

34 Gowing, *Common Bodies*, pp. 48, 50.

35 Jens Lachmund, *Der abgehorchte Körper: zur historischen Soziologie der medizinischen Untersuchung* (Opladen, 1997), pp. 52–100.

36 Erwin H. Ackerknecht, *Medicine at the Paris Hospital 1774–1848* (Baltimore, 1967).

37 Michel Foucault, *The Birth of the Clinic. An Archaeology of Medical Perception* (New York, [1973] 1994), pp. 124–148.

38 Ibid., p. xviii.

39 Nicolas D. Jewson, 'The Disappearance of the Sick-man from Medical Cosmology, 1770–1870', *Sociology*, 10:2 (1976), pp. 225–244; Ian Miller, *Medical History* (London, 2018), pp. 108–114.

40 Edward Shorter, *A History of Psychiatry. From the Era of the Asylum to the Age of Prozac* (New York, 1997), pp. 69–112.

41 Fay Bound Alberti, *Matters of the Heart: History, Medicine, and Emotion* (Oxford, 2010), pp. 6–9.

42 Fernando Vidal, 'Brainhood, Anthropological Figure of Modernity', *History of the Human Sciences*, 22:1 (2009), pp. 5–36.

43 Wolfgang Schivelbusch, *The Railway Journey. The Industrialization of Time and Space in the Nineteenth Century* (Leamington Spa, [1977] 1986), pp. 134–149.

44 Peter Leese, *Shell Shock: Traumatic Neurosis and the British Soldiers of the First World War* (New York, 2002).

45 Willemijn Ruberg, 'Trauma, Body and Mind. Forensic Medicine in Nineteenth-Century Dutch Rape Cases', *Journal of the History of Sexuality*, 22:1 (2013), pp. 85–104.

46 Georges Vigarello, *Rape: A History from 1860 to the Present Day* (London, 2007), pp. 130, 161, 197.

47 Monica H. Green, 'Bodily Essences. Bodies as Categories of Difference', in Kalof, ed., *A Cultural History of the Human Body*, Part 2, 'In the Medieval Age', pp. 159–160.

48 Merlijn Schoonenboom, '"Mag Ik U Mijn vriend Noemen?". De Fysiognomische Correspondentie van Johann Kaspar Lavater', *Krisis*, 3 (2003), p. 35.

49 Roger Cooter, *The Cultural Meaning of Popular Science: Phrenology and the Organization of Consent in Nineteenth-Century Britain* (Cambridge, 1984).

50 Joseph Dumit, *Picturing Personhood: Brain Scans and Biomedical Identity* (Princeton, 2003), pp. 7, 160; see also Fenneke Sysling, 'Science and Self-Assessment: Phrenological Charts 1840–1940', *The British Journal for the History of Science*, 51:2 (2018), pp. 261–280.

51 Simon Cole, *Suspect Identities. A History of Fingerprinting and Criminal Identification* (Harvard, 2002), pp. 5, 100.

52 David G. Horn, *The Criminal Body. Lombroso and the Anatomy of Deviance* (New York, 2003), pp. 1–27.

53 Jerrold Seigel, *The Idea of the Self. Thought and Experience in Western Europe since the Seventeenth Century* (Cambridge, 2005); Charles Taylor, *Sources of the Self: The Making of the Modern Identity* (Cambridge, 1989); Raymond Martin and John Barresi, *The Rise and Fall of Soul and Self: An Intellectual History of Personal Identity* (New York, 2008); Roy Porter, 'Introduction', in Idem, ed., *Rewriting the Self. Histories from the Renaissance to the Present* (London, 1997), p. 1.

54 Dror Wahrman, *The Making of the Modern Self. Identity and Culture in Eighteenth-Century England* (New Haven, CT, 2004).

55 Nazife Bashar, 'Rape in England Between 1550 and 1700', in The London Feminist History Group, ed., *The Sexual Dynamics of History. Men's Power, Women's Resistance* (London, 1983), p. 41; Miranda Chaytor, 'Husbandry: Narratives of Rape in the Seventeenth Century', *Gender and History*, 7:3 (1995), pp. 395–396; Garthine Walker, 'Rereading Rape and Sexual Violence in Early Modern England', *Gender and History*, 10:1 (1998), p. 19.

56 Vigarello, *Rape*, pp. 130, 161, 197.

57 George L. Mosse, *The Image of Man. The Creation of Modern Masculinity* (New York, 1996).

58 Charlotte Macdonald, 'Body and Self: Learning to be Modern in 1920s–1930s Britain', *Women's History Review*, 22:2 (2013), p. 272.

59 Ibid., p. 275.

60 Christopher E. Forth, 'The Qualities of Fat: Bodies, History, and Materiality', *Journal of Material Culture*, 18:2 (2013), p. 136; see also Christopher E. Forth, *Fat. A Cultural History of the Stuff of Life* (London, 2019).

61 Sander L. Gilman, *Obesity: The Biography* (Oxford, 2010); Peter Stearns, *Fat History: Bodies and Beauty in the Modern West* (New York, [1997] 2012). For an overview of the literature see: Nina Mackert, 'Writing the History of Fat Agency', *Body Politics*, 3:5 (2015), pp. 15–18.

62 Joan Jacobs Brumberg, *Fasting Girls. The History of Anorexia Nervosa* (New York, [1988] 2000), pp. 230–231.

63 Christopher E. Forth, 'On Fat and Fattening: Agency, Materiality and Animality in the History of Corpulence', *Body Politics*, 3:5 (2015), p. 66.

64 Ibid., p. 67.

65 Peter Stearns, *Fat History: Bodies and Beauty in the Modern West* (New York, [1997] 2012).

66 Susan Bordo, *Unbearable Weight. Feminism, Western Culture and the Body* (Berkeley, CA, 1993), p. 116 dates this attack already to an earlier Victorian ideology; Brumberg, *Fasting Girls*, pp. 236–246.

▶ 2 The Modern Body, Discipline, and Agency

1 Norbert Elias, *The Civilizing Process. Sociogenetic and Psychogenetic Investigations*, ed. by Eric Dunning, Johan Goudsblom and Stephen Mennell, translated by Edmund Jephcott (rev. ed. Oxford, [1939] 2000), p. 139.

2 Norbert Elias, *The Court Society*, translated by Edmund Jephcott (Oxford, 1983), pp. 231–232.

3 Shilling, *The Body & Social Theory*, p. 162.

4 Ibid., p. 175.

5 Ibid., p. 161.

6 Mike Atkinson, 'Norbert Elias and the Body', in Bryan S. Turner, ed., *Routledge Handbook of Body Studies* (London, 2012), p. 53.

7 Shilling, *The Body & Social Theory*, p. 182.

8 Barbara Rosenwein, 'Worrying about Emotions in History', *The American Historical Review*, 107:3 (2002), p. 841.

9 Shilling, *The Body & Social Theory*, p. 183.

10 Ibid., p. 185.

11 Anna Bryson, *From Courtesy to Civility: Changing Codes of Conduct in Early Modern England* (New York, 1998), pp. 7, 11, 278–279.

12 Shilling, *The Body & Social Theory*, pp. 165–166.

13 Norbert Elias, 'Introduction', in Norbert Elias and Eric Dunning, eds, *Quest for Excitement: Sport and Leisure in the Civilizing Process* (Oxford, 1986), p. 21.

14 Rosenwein, 'Worrying about Emotions in History', pp. 835–837.

15 E.P. Thompson, 'Time, Work-Discipline and Industrial Capitalism', *Past and Present*, 38:1 (1967), p. 90.

16 Michel Foucault, *Discipline and Punish. The Birth of the Prison*, translated by Alan Sheridan, 2nd edn (New York, [1977] 1995), p. 26.
17 Nikolas Rose, 'The Politics of Life Itself', *Theory, Culture and Society*, 18:6 (2001), pp. 1–30.
18 Foucault, *Discipline and Punish*, p. 136.
19 Susan Bordo, *Unbearable Weight. Feminism, Western Culture and the Body* (Berkeley, 1993), p. 112.
20 Ibid., p. 130.
21 Ibid., p. 186.
22 Colin Jones and Roy Porter, 'Introduction', in Idem, eds, *Reassessing Foucault: Power, Medicine and the Body* (London, 1994), p. 4.
23 Lois McNay, *Foucault and Feminism: Power, Gender and the Self* (Cambridge, 1992), p. 3.
24 Jones and Porter, 'Introduction', p. 3.
25 Irene Diamond and Lee Quinby, 'Introduction', in Idem, eds, *Feminism and Foucault: Reflections on Resistance* (Boston, MA, 1988), p. x.
26 Jana Sawicki, *Disciplining Foucault. Feminism, Power, and the Body* (New York, 1991), pp. 1–15; McNay, *Foucault and Feminism*, p. 4.
27 Michel Foucault, 'Technologies of the Self', in Luther Martin and Patrick H. Hutton, eds, *Technologies of the Self. A Seminar with Michel Foucault* (Amherst, 1988), p. 18.
28 Ciara Breathnach and Elaine Farrell, '"Indelible Characters". Tattoos, Power and the Late Nineteenth Century Irish Convict Body', *Cultural and Social History*, 12:2 (2015), pp. 235–254.
29 Lois McNay, 'Gender, Habitus and the Field. Pierre Bourdieu and the Limits of Reflexivity', *Theory, Culture and Society*, 16:1 (1999), p. 96.
30 Edward W. Said, *Orientalism* (London, 1978).
31 Robbie McVeigh and Bill Rolston, 'Civilising the Irish', *Race & Class*, 51:1 (2009), pp. 5–7.
32 Ibid., p. 12.
33 Margrit Pernau and Helge Jorheim, 'Introduction', in Idem et al., eds, *Civilizing Emotions. Concepts in Nineteenth-Century Asia and Europe* (Oxford, 2015), p. 9.
34 Ornella Moscucci, *The Science of Woman. Gynaecology and Gender in England, 1800–1929* (Cambridge, 1990), pp. 4, 24–27.
35 Laura Briggs, 'The Race of Hysteria: "Overcivilization" and the "Savage" Woman in Late Nineteenth-Century Obstetrics and Gynecology', *American Quarterly*, 52:2 (2000), p. 250.

36 Ibid., p. 262.
37 Anupama Rao and Steven Pierce, 'Discipline and the Other Body. Humanitarianism, Violence, and the Colonial Exception', in Steven Pierce and Anupama Rao, eds, *Discipline and the Other Body* (Durham, NC, 2006) p. 21.
38 Dorothy Ko, *Cinderella's Sisters: A Revisionist History of Footbinding* (Berkeley, 2005).
39 Dorothy Ko, 'Footbinding and Anti-Footbinding in China. The Subject of Pain in the Nineteenth and Early Twentieth Centuries', in Pierce and Anupama, eds, *Discipline and the Other Body*, p. 216.
40 Ko, *Cinderella's Sisters*, p. 13.
41 Gayatri Chakravorty Spivak, 'Can the Subaltern Speak?', in Laura Chrisman and Patrick Williams, eds, *Colonial Discourse and Post-Colonial Theory: A Reader* (New York, 1993), p. 93.
42 Joanne Entwistle, *The Fashioned Body. Fashion, Dress and Modern Social Theory* (Cambridge, [2000] 2006), pp. 161–163; 195–200.
43 Joan Jacobs Brumberg, *The Body Project. An Intimate History of American Girls* (New York, [1997] 1998), p. 70.
44 Ibid., p. 70.
45 Ibid., pp. 98–99.
46 Ibid., pp. 68–69.
47 Annelie Ramsbrock, *The Science of Beauty. Culture and Cosmetics in Modern Germany, 1750–1930*, translated by David Burnett (Basingstoke, 2015).
48 Rebecca M. Herzig, *Plucked. A History of Hair Removal* (New York, 2015), p. 77.
49 Ibid., pp. 187–191.
50 Stearns, *Fat History*, p. 249.
51 Lynn M. Thomas, 'Historicising Agency', *Gender & History*, 28:2 (2016), pp. 325–326.
52 Ibid., p. 326.
53 Ibid., p. 332.
54 Ibid.
55 Forth, 'On Fat and Fattening', pp. 51–74.
56 Boston Women's Health Collective, *Women and their Bodies. A Course* (1970), p. 4, original typescript, found at www.ourbodiesourselves.org/cms/assets/uploads/2014/04/Women-and-Their-Bodies-1970.pdf [accessed 18 Dec.2018].
57 Kathy Davis, *The Making of Our Bodies, Ourselves: How Feminism Travels Across Borders* (Durham, NC, 2007).

58 Stephanie M.H. Camp, 'Black is Beautiful: An American History', *The Journal of Southern History*, 81:3 (2015), pp. 675–690.
59 Jerry Alan Winter, 'The Development of the Disability Rights Movement as a Social Problem Solver', *Disability Studies Quarterly*, 23:1 (2003), pp. 33–61.
60 Alicia Ouellette, 'Hearing the Deaf: Cochlear Implants, the Deaf Community, and Bioethical Analysis', *Valparaiso University Law Review*, 45:3 (2011), pp. 1247–1270.
61 Nora Kreuzenbeck, 'Nothing to Lose: Fat Acceptance-Strategien und Agency als Widerstand und Unterwerfung in den USA von der Mitte der 1960er bis in die frühen 1980er Jahre', *Body Politics*, 3:5 (2015), pp. 111–134.
62 Lois McNay, *Gender and Agency: Reconfiguring the Subject in Feminist and Social Theory* (Cambridge, 2000), p. 2.

▶ 3 The Social Construction of the Body and Disease

1 Shilling, *The Body & Social Theory*, p. 75.
2 Darin Weinberg, *Contemporary Social Constructionism* (Philadelphia, 2014), p. 86.
3 Claude Lévi-Strauss, *Structural Anthropology*, translated by Claire Jacobson and Brooke Grundfest Schoepf (New York, 1963), p. 257.
4 Mary Douglas, *Purity and Danger. An Analysis of Concepts of Pollution and Taboo* (London, [1966] 2008), pp. 149–150.
5 E.R. Leach, 'Magical Hair', *The Journal of the Royal Anthropological Institute of Great Britain and Ireland*, 88:2 (1958), p. 157.
6 Douglas, *Purity and Danger*, p. 152.
7 Thomas Buckley and Alma Gottlieb, 'A Critical Appraisal of Theories of Menstrual Symbolism', in Thomas Buckley and Alma Gottlieb, eds, *Blood Magic. The Anthropology of Menstruation* (Berkeley, 1988), pp. 3–50.
8 Douglas, *Purity and Danger*, p. 187.
9 Willemijn Ruberg, 'The Tactics of Menstruation in Dutch Cases of Sexual Assault and Infanticide, 1750–1920', *Journal of Women's History*, 25:3 (2013), pp. 29–30.
10 Michael Stolberg, 'An Unmanly Vice: Self-Pollution, Anxiety, and the Body in the Eighteenth Century', *Social History of Medicine*, 13:1 (2000), p. 20.
11 Alison Bashford, *Purity and Pollution. Gender, Embodiment and Victorian Medicine* (New York, 1998).

12 Susan Sontag, *Illness as Metaphor and AIDS and Its Metaphors* (New York, [1978] 1988/1989), pp. 64–66.

13 Ibid., p. 7.

14 Emily Martin, 'The Egg and the Sperm: How Science has Constructed a Romance Based on Stereotypical Male-Female Roles', *Signs: Journal of Women in Culture and Society*, 16:3 (1991), p. 487.

15 Ibid., p. 491.

16 Ibid., p. 500.

17 Miller, *Medical History*, pp. 39–42.

18 Ibid., p. 39.

19 Roger Cooter and Claudia Stein, 'Introduction', in Idem, eds, *The History of Medicine. Critical Concepts in Historical Studies*, part 1 'Ancient and Medieval Medicine' (London, 2016), pp. 1–32; Mary Fissell, 'Making Meaning from the Margins: The New Cultural History of Medicine', in John Harley Warner and Frank Huisman, eds, *Locating Medical History: Stories and their Meanings* (Baltimore, 2004), pp. 364–389.

20 Charles E. Rosenberg, 'Introduction. Framing Disease: Illness, Society and History', in Charles E. Rosenberg and Janet Golden, eds, *Framing Disease. Studies in Cultural History*, 2nd edn (New Brunswick, NJ, [1992] 1997), p. xviii.

21 Ibid., pp. xiv–xv.

22 Henrice Altink, 'Editorial: From the Local to the Global: Fifty Years of Historical Research on Tuberculosis', *Medical History*, 59:1 (2015), p. 3.

23 Barron H. Lerner, 'From Careless Consumptives to Recalcitrant Patients: The Historical Construction of Noncompliance', *Social Science & Medicine*, 45:9 (1997), p. 1426.

24 Paul H. Mason et al., 'Social, Historical and Cultural Dimensions of Tuberculosis', *Journal of Biosocial Science*, 48:2 (2016), p. 215.

25 Katherine Ott, *Fevered Lives: Tuberculosis in American Culture Since 1870* (Cambridge, MA, 1996), p. 4.

26 Ibid., p. 1.

27 Ibid., p. 7.

28 Mark Micale, 'Charcot and the Idea of Hysteria in the Male: Gender, Mental Science, and Medical Diagnosis in Late Nineteenth-Century France', *Medical History*, 34 (1990), p. 366; Andrew Scull, *Hysteria. The Disturbing History* (Oxford, [2009] 2011), p. 25.

29 Micale, 'Charcot', p. 393.

30 Micale, 'Charcot', pp. 406–408; see also Mark Micale, *Hysterical Men: The Hidden History of Male Nervous Illness* (Cambridge, MA, 2008).

31 Mark Micale, 'On the "Disappearance" of Hysteria: A Study in the Clinical Deconstruction of a Diagnosis', *Isis*, 84:3 (1993), pp. 496–526.

32 Anthony Feinstein, 'Conversion Disorder: Advances in Our Understanding', *CMAJ*, 183:8 (2011), pp. 915–920; Jon Stone et al., 'The Disappearance of Hysteria: Historical Mystery or Illusion?', *Journal of the Royal Society of Medicine*, 101:1 (2008), pp. 12–18.

33 Carroll Smith-Rosenberg, 'The Hysterical Woman: Sex Roles and the Role Conflict in Nineteenth Century America', *Social Research*, 39:4 (1972), p. 678.

34 Brumberg, *Fasting Girls*, pp. 43–44.

35 Ibid., pp. 109–127.

36 Ibid., pp. 26–44.

37 Bordo, *Unbearable Weight*, p. 69.

38 Rosemarie Garland-Thomson, 'Integrating Disability, Transforming Feminist Theory', *NWSA Journal*, 14:3 (2002), pp. 1–32; Catherine J. Kudlick, 'Disability History: Why We Need Another "Other"', *American Historical Review*, 108:3 (2003), pp. 763–793.

39 Lennard J. Davis, 'Constructing Normalcy: The Bell Curve, the Novel, and the Invention of the Disabled Body in the Nineteenth Century', in Idem, ed., *The Disability Studies Reader* (New York, 1997), pp. 9–29.

40 Paul K. Longmore and David Goldberger, 'The League of the Physically Handicapped and the Great Depression, A Case Study in the New Disability History', *The Journal of American History*, 87:3 (2000), pp. 888–922.

41 Garland-Thomson, 'Integrating Disability, Transforming Feminist Theory', p. 3.

42 Sadiah Qureshi, 'Displaying Sara Baartman, the "Hottentot Venus"', *History of Science*, 42 (2004), pp. 233–257.

43 Garland-Thomson, 'Integrating Disability, Transforming Feminist Theory', p. 7.

44 Douglas C. Baynton, 'Disability and the Justification of Inequality in American History', in Paul K. Longmore and Lauri Umansky, eds, *The New Disability History. American Perspectives* (New York, 2001), pp. 33–57.

45 Janine Owens, 'Exploring the Critiques of the Social Model of Disability: The Transformative Possibility of Arendt's Notion of Power', *Sociology of Health and Illness*, 37:3 (2015), p. 388.

46 Ian Hacking, *The Social Construction of What?* (Cambridge, MA, [1999] 2000), p. 6.

47 Ibid., pp. 16–17.

48 Ibid., p. 11.

49 Ibid., p. 105.

50 Ludmilla Jordanova, 'The Social Construction of Medical Knowledge', *Social History of Medicine*, 8:3 (1995), p. 377.

51 Ibid., p. 368.

52 Weinberg, *Contemporary Social Constructionism*, pp. 81–100.

53 Jordanova, 'The Social Construction of Medical Knowledge', p. 368.

54 Ibid., p. 375.

55 Jeff Coulter, 'Ian Hacking on Constructionism', *Science, Technology & Human Values*, 26:1 (2001), pp. 82–86.

▶ 4 The Body, Gender, and Sexuality

1 Joan W. Scott, 'Gender: A Useful Category of Analysis', *American Historical Review*, 91:5 (1986), pp. 1053–1075.

2 Gayle Rubin, 'The Traffic in Women: Notes on the "Political Economy" of Sex', in Rayna R. Reiter, ed., *Toward an Anthropology of Women* (New York, 1975), p. 165.

3 Thomas Laqueur, *Making Sex: Body and Gender from the Greeks to Freud* (Cambridge, MA, [1990] 1992), p. 107.

4 Ibid.

5 Londa Schiebinger,'Skeletons in the Closet: The First Illustrations of the Female Skeleton in Eighteenth-Century Anatomy', *Representations*, 14 (1986), pp. 42–82.

6 Joan Cadden, *Meanings of Sex Difference in the Middle Ages: Medicine, Science and Culture* (Cambridge, 1993); Katharine Park and Robert Nye, 'Destiny is Anatomy', *New Republic*, 7 (18 Feb. 1991), p. 54; Helen King, *Hippocrates' Woman: Reading the Female Body in Ancient Greece* (London, 1998), p. 11; Helen King, *The One-Sex Body on Trial: The Classical and Early Modern Evidence* (Farnham, 2014).

7 Michael Stolberg, 'A Woman Down to Her Bones. The Anatomy of Sexual Difference in the Sixteenth and Early Seventeenth Centuries', *Isis*, 94:2 (2003), pp. 274–299; for Laqueur's reply see: Thomas Laqueur, 'Sex in the Flesh', *Isis*, 94:2 (2003), pp. 300–306.

8 Gowing, *Common Bodies*, pp. 2–4; Fissell, *Vernacular Bodies*, pp. 12–13.

9 Wendy D. Churchill, 'The Medical Practice of the Sexed Body: Women, Men and Disease in Britain, circa 1600–1740', *Social History of Medicine*, 18:1 (2005), pp. 3–22.

10 Cathy McClive, 'Masculinity on Trial: Penises, Hermaphrodites and the Uncertain Male Body in Early Modern France', *History Workshop Journal*, 68 (2009), p. 45.

11 Ibid., p. 65.

12 Moscucci, *The Science of Woman*, p. 33.

13 Ibid., p. 28.

14 Mary Poovey, '"Scenes of an Indelicate Character": The Medical "Treatment" of Victorian Women', *Representations*, 14 (1986), pp. 145–146.

15 Lisa Wynne Smith, 'The Body Embarrassed? Rethinking the Leaky Male Body in Eighteenth-Century England and France', *Gender & History*, 23:1 (2010), pp. 26–46.

16 Michael Stolberg, 'Menstruation and Sexual Difference in Early Modern Medicine', in Andrew Shail and Gillian Howie, eds, *Menstruation. A Cultural History* (Basingstoke, 2005), pp. 90–101, 99.

17 Moscucci, *The Science of Woman*, pp. 25, 34.

18 Lidy Schoon, *De Gynaecologie als Belichaming van Vrouwen. Verloskunde en Gynaecologie 1840–1920* (Zutphen, 1995), pp. 166–178; Julie-Marie Strange, 'Menstrual Fictions: Languages of Medicine and Menstruation, c. 1850–1930', *Women's History Review*, 9:3 (2000), p. 618.

19 Nelly Oudshoorn, *Beyond the Natural Body. An Archeology of Sex Hormones* (London, 1994), p. 39.

20 Ibid., pp. 145–147.

21 Anne Fausto-Sterling, *Sexing the Body. Gender Politics and the Construction of Sexuality* (New York, 2000), pp. 45–77.

22 Ibid., p. 3.

23 Mary Wollstonecraft, *A Vindication of the Rights of Women* (Oxford, [1792] 2008), p. 112.

24 Simone de Beauvoir, *The Second Sex*, translated by Constance Borde and Sheila Malovany-Chevallier (London, [1949] 2009), p. 293.

25 Ibid., p. 42.

26 Ibid., p. 552.

27 Ibid., p. 409.

28 Toril Moi, *Simone de Beauvoir. The Making of an Intellectual Woman*, 2nd edn (Oxford, [1994] 2008), p. 190.

29 Rosemarie Putnam Tong, *Feminist Thought. A More Comprehensive Introduction*, 2nd edn (Boulder, CO, 1988), p. 125.

30 Moi, *Simone de Beauvoir*, p. 191.

31 Harry Oosterhuis, *Stepchildren of Nature: Krafft-Ebing, Psychiatry and the Making of Sexual Identity* (Chicago, 2000); Lucy Bland and Laura Doan, *Sexology in Culture: Labelling Bodies and Desires* (Chicago, 1998).

32 Michel Foucault, *The History of Sexuality*, part 1 'The Will to Knowledge' (London, [1976] 1998).

33 Laura Doan, *Disturbing Practices. History, Sexuality, and Women's Experience of Modern War* (Chicago, 2013), p. 6.

34 Theo van der Meer, 'Sodomy and its Discontents: Discourse, Desire and the Rise of a Same-Sex Proto Something in the Early Modern Dutch Republic', *Historical Reflections*, 33:1 (2007), p. 55.

35 Ibid., pp. 41–67.

36 Nikki Sullivan, *A Critical Introduction to Queer Theory* (New York, [2003] 2006).

37 David Halperin, *Saint Foucault: Towards a Gay Hagiography* (Oxford, 1995), p. 62, emphasis in original.

38 Judith Butler, *Gender Trouble. Feminism and the Subversion of Identity* (New York, [1990] 1999), p. 173, emphasis in original.

39 Foucault, *The History of Sexuality*, part 1 'The Will to Knowledge', p. 154.

40 Butler, *Gender Trouble*, p. 31.

41 Judith Butler, *Bodies that Matter: On the Discursive Limits of 'Sex'* (London, 1993).

42 Judith Butler, Peter Osborne and Lynne Segal, 'Gender as Performance: An Interview with Judith Butler', *Radical Philosophy*, 67 (1994), pp. 32–37.

43 Ibid., p. 34.

44 Samuel A. Chambers, '"Sex" and the Problem of the Body: Reconstructing Judith Butler's Theory of Sex/Gender', *Body & Society*, 13:4 (2007), p. 64.

45 Fiona Webster, 'The Politics of Sex and Gender: Benhabib and Butler Debate Subjectivity', *Hypatia*, 15:1 (2000), pp. 1–22.

46 In the late 1980s the term 'transgender' came to be used instead of the more medical term 'transsexual'.

47 Sullivan, *A Critical Introduction to Queer Theory*, p. 112.

48 Ibid., pp. 105–110.

49 Ibid., pp. 99–118.

50 Jonathan Ned Katz, *The Invention of Heterosexuality* (Chicago, 1995).

51 H.G. Cocks, 'Modernity and the Self in the History of Sexuality', *The Historical Journal*, 49:4 (2006), pp. 1219–1222.

52 Jeanne Boydston, 'Gender as a Question of Historical Analysis', *Gender and History*, 20:3 (2008), p. 574.

53 Oyèrónké Oyewúmí, 'Visualizing the Body: Western Theories and African Subjects', in Oyèrónké Oyewúmí, ed., *African Gender Studies: A Reader* (New York, 2005), p. 11, quoted in Boydston, 'Gender as a Question of Historical Analysis', p. 580 note 24.

54 Sue-Ellen Jacobs, Wesley Thomas and Sabine Lang, eds, *Two-Spirit People: Native American Gender Identity, Sexuality, and Spirituality* (Urbana, 1997).

55 Nancy Shoemaker, 'Categories', in Idem, ed., *Clearing a Path: Theorizing the Past in Native American Cultures* (London, 2002), p. 59, quoted in Boyston, 'Gender as a Question of Historical Analysis', p. 582, note 53.

56 Boydston, 'Gender as a Question of Historical Analysis', pp. 576–577.

57 Ivan Crozier, '(De-)constructing Sexual Kinds since 1750', in Toulalan and Fischer, *The Routledge History of Sex and the Body*, p. 142. See also Harry Oosterhuis, 'Sexual Modernity in the Works of Richard von Krafft-Ebing and Albert Moll', *Medical History*, 56 (2012), p. 138.

58 Crozier, '(De-)constructing Sexual Kinds Since 1750', p. 147.

▶ **5 Experiencing the Body**

1 Kathleen Canning, 'The Body as Method? Reflections on the Place of the Body in Gender History', *Gender & History*, 11:3 (1999), p. 501; Shilling, *The Body & Social Theory*, p. 84, 243.

2 Drew Leder, 'A Tale of Two Bodies: The Cartesian Corpse and the Lived Body', in Donn Welton, ed., *Body and Flesh, A Philosophical Reader* (Malden, MA, 1998), pp. 122–124.

3 Turner, *The Body & Society*, p. 245.

4 Canning, 'The Body as Method?', p. 505.

5 Janine Pierret, 'The Illness Experience: State of Knowledge and Perspectives for Research', *Sociology of Health & Illness*, 25 (2003), pp. 4–6.

6 Roy Porter, 'The Patient's View: Doing Medical History from Below', *Theory and Society*, 14:2 (1985), pp. 175–198.

7 Joan Scott, 'The Evidence of Experience', *Critical Inquiry*, 17:4 (1991), pp. 773–797.

8 Jenny Slatman, 'Inleiding' in Maurice Merleau-Ponty, ed., *De Wereld Waarnemen*, translated by Jenny Slatman (Amsterdam, 2003), p. 11.

9 Maurice Merleau-Ponty, *Phenomenology of Perception*, translated by Colin Smith (London, [1945]) part I.

10 Nick Crossley, 'Phenomenology and the Body', in Turner, ed., *Routledge Handbook of Body Studies*, p. 135.

11 Merleau-Ponty, *Phenomenology of Perception*, p. 106.

12 Leder, 'A Tale of Two Bodies: The Cartesian Corpse and the Lived Body', p. 124.

13 Elizabeth Grosz, *Volatile Bodies. Toward a Corporeal Feminism* (Bloomington, 1994), p. 95.

14 David Woodruff Smith, 'Phenomenology', in Edward N. Zalta, ed., *The Stanford Encyclopedia of Philosophy* (Winter 2016 Edition), https://plato. stanford.edu/archives/win2016/entries/phenomenology/ (accessed 18 Dec. 2018).

15 Maurice Merleau-Ponty, *The Primacy of Perception*, ed. James M. Edie (Evanston, 1964), p. 5.

16 Iris Marion Young, 'Throwing like a Girl: A Phenomenology of Feminine Body Comportment Motility and Spatiality', *Human Studies*, 3 (1980), p. 143.

17 Ibid., p. 145.

18 Ibid., p. 152.

19 David Macey, 'Fanon, Phenomenology, Race', *Radical Philosophy*, 95 (1999), pp. 8–14.

20 Cynthia R. Nielsen, 'Resistance Through Re-narration: Fanon on Deconstructing Racialized Subjectivities', *African Identities*, 9:4 (2011), p. 364.

21 Frantz Fanon, *Black Skin, White Masks*, translated by Richard Philcox (New York, [1952] 2008), p. 92.

22 Ibid., p. 95, emphasis in original.

23 Ibid., p. 91.

24 Teresa de Lauretis, 'Difference Embodied: Reflections on *Black Skin, White Masks*', *Parallax*, 8:2 (2002), p. 57.

25 Sara Ahmed, 'A Phenomenology of Whiteness', *Feminist Theory*, 8:2 (2007), p. 153.

26 Nielsen, 'Resistance Through Re-narration', p. 368.

27 Ahmed, 'A Phenomenology of Whiteness', p. 161.

28 Fanon, *Black Skin, White Masks*, pp. 90–92.

29 de Lauretis, 'Difference Embodied', p. 58.

30 Jeremy Weate, 'Fanon, Merleau-Ponty and the Difference of Phenomenology', in R. Bernasconi, ed., *Race* (Oxford, 2000), p. 175.

31 Nielsen, 'Resistance Through Re-narration', p. 373.

32 Ahmed, 'A Phenomenology of Whiteness', p. 150.

33 Linda Martín Alcoff, 'Toward a Phenomenology of Racial Embodiment', in Bernasconi, ed., *Race*, pp. 271–272.

34 Barbara Duden, *The Woman Beneath the Skin. A Doctor's Patients in Eighteenth-Century Germany*, translated by Thomas Dunlap (Cambridge, MA, [1987] 1991), p. vii.

35 Ibid., p. 44.

36 Isabel V. Hull, 'The Body as Historical Experience. Review of Recent Works by Barbara Duden', *Central European History*, 28 (1995), p. 77.

37 Duden, *The Woman Beneath the Skin*, pp. 41–44.

38 Hull, 'The Body as Historical Experience', p. 75.

39 Duden, *The Woman Beneath the Skin*, pp. vii–viii.

40 Hull, 'The Body as Historical Experience', pp. 76–78.

41 Bruce R. Smith, 'Premodern Sexualities', *PMLA*, 115:3 (2000), p. 325. See also Bruce R. Smith, *Phenomenal Shakespeare* (Malden, MA, 2010).

42 Kevin Curran and James Kearney, 'Introduction', special issue on 'Shakespeare and Phenomenology', *Criticism*, 54:3 (2012), p. 354.

43 Gail Kern Paster, *Humoring the Body: Emotions and the Shakespearean Stage* (Chicago, 2010), pp. 5, 26.

44 Ibid., p. 22.

45 Ibid., p. 8.

46 Ibid., pp. 19, 40–41.

47 Séverine Pilloud and Micheline Louis-Courvoisier, 'The Intimate Experience of the Body in the Eighteenth Century: Between Interiority and Exteriority', *Medical History*, 47 (2003), p. 454. See also Gudrun Piller, 'Krankheit schreiben. Körper und Sprache im Selbstzeugnis von Margarethe E. Milow-Hudtwalcker (1748–1794)', *Historische Anthropologie*, 7 (1999), pp. 212–235.

48 Joanna Bourke, *The Story of Pain. From Prayer to Painkillers* (Oxford, 2014), pp. 4–5.

49 Ibid., pp. 6–8.

50 Ibid., pp. 16–18.

51 Joanna Bourke, 'Pain: Metaphor, Body, and Culture in Anglo-American Societies Between the Eighteenth and Twentieth Centuries', *Rethinking History*, 18:4 (2014), pp. 476–477.

52 Ibid., p. 481.
53 Ibid., pp. 486–487.
54 Ibid., p. 488.
55 Ibid., pp. 488–493.
56 Ibid., pp. 488, 494–495.
57 Lindon Barrett, 'African-American Slave Narratives: Literacy, the Body, Authority', *American Literary History*, 7:3 (1995), pp. 420, 426.
58 Katherine Fishburn, *The Problem of Embodiment in Early African American Narrative* (Westport, CT, 1997), p. xii.
59 Ibid., p. 35.
60 Ibid., p. 58.
61 Ibid., pp. 61–62.
62 Ibid., pp. 96–97.
63 Marcel Mauss, 'Body Techniques', in Jonathan Crary and Sanford Kwinter, eds, *Incorporations. Zone 6* (New York, 1992), pp. 455–477.
64 C. Jason Throop and Keith M. Murphy, 'Bourdieu and Phenomenology. A Critical Assessment', *Anthropological Theory*, 2:2 (2002), pp. 189–191.
65 Pierre Bourdieu, *The Logic of Practice*, translated by R. Nice (Cambridge, 1992), p. 53.
66 Craig Calhoun, 'Pierre Bourdieu', in George Ritzer, ed., *The Blackwell Companion to Major Social Theorists* (Oxford, 2000), p. 712.
67 Herman Roodenburg, *The Eloquence of the Body. Perspectives on Gesture in the Dutch Republic* (Zwolle, 2001), p. 21.
68 Shilling, *The Body & Social Theory*, p. 246.
69 Simon Gunn, *History and Cultural Theory* (Harlow, 2006), pp. 76–78.
70 Rosenwein, 'Worrying About Emotions in History', p. 837.
71 Josephine Hoegaerts and Tine van Osselaer, 'De Lichamelijkheid van Emoties. Een Introductie', *Tijdschrift voor Geschiedenis*, 126:4 (2013), pp. 452–465.
72 Monique Scheer, 'Are Emotions a Kind of Practice (and Is That What Makes Them Have a History)? A Bourdieuian Approach to Understanding Emotion', *History and Theory*, 51 (2012), p. 193.
73 Ibid., pp. 209–210.
74 Ibid., pp. 217–218.
75 Roodenburg, *The Eloquence of the Body*, p. 94.
76 Paul Connerton, *How Societies Remember* (Cambridge, 1989).
77 Roodenburg, *The Eloquence of the Body*, pp. 19–23.
78 Ibid., pp. 23–25.

79 McNay, 'Gender, Habitus and the Field', pp. 95, 101.

80 Shilling, *The Body & Social Theory*, p. 157.

81 Garthine Walker, 'Psychoanalysis and History', in Stefan Berger, Heiko Feldner and Kevin Passmore, eds, *Writing History. Theory & Practice* (London, 2003), pp. 141–142, 151.

82 Lyndal Roper, 'Witchcraft and Fantasy in Early Modern Germany', *History Workshop Journal*, 32 (1991), p. 27.

83 Ibid., p. 22.

84 Ibid., p. 31.

85 Lyndal Roper, *Oedipus and the Devil. Witchcraft, Sexuality and Religion in Early Modern Europe* (London, 1994), p. 22.

86 Ibid., p. 3.

87 Laura Lee Downs, *Writing Gender History* (London, 2004), p. 166.

88 Roper, *Oedipus and the Devil*, pp. 9, 22.

89 Turner, *The Body & Society*, p. 52; Shilling, *The Body & Social Theory*, p. 245.

90 Paul Münch, 'Einleitung', in Idem, ed., *'Erfahrung' als Kategorie der Frühneuzeitgeschichte* (Munich, 2001) p. 18.

91 Bruce R. Smith, 'Phenomophobia, or Who's afraid of Merleau-Ponty?', *Criticism*, 54:3 (2012), pp. 480–481.

92 Moira Gatens, *Imaginary Bodies. Ethics, Power and Corporeality* (New York, 1996), p. viii.

▶ 6 Materialist Approaches to the Body

1 Diana Coole and Samantha Frost, 'Introducing the New Materialism', in Idem, ed., *New Materialisms: Ontology, Agency, Politics* (Durham, 2010), p. 6.

2 Donna Haraway, 'A Cyborg Manifesto: Science, Technology, and Socialist-Feminism in the Late Twentieth Century', in Idem, ed., *Simians, Cyborgs and Women: The Reinvention of Nature* (New York, [1985] 1991), p. 150.

3 Ibid., p. 177.

4 Daniel Lord Smail, *On Deep History and the Brain* (Berkeley, CA, 2007), p. 114.

5 Ibid., p. 117.

6 Ibid., p. 183.

7 Ibid., p. 185.

8 Ibid., p. 188.

9 Anne Fausto-Sterling, 'The Bare Bones of Sex: Part 1 – Sex and Gender', *Signs*, 30:2 (2005), pp. 1491–1527. See also Idem, 'The Bare Bones of Race', *Social Studies of Science*, 38:5 (2008), pp. 657–694.

10 Dror Wahrman, 'Change and the Corporeal in Seventeenth- and Eighteenth-Century Gender History: Or, Can Cultural History be Rigorous?', *Gender & History*, 20:3 (2008), p. 601.

11 Fausto-Sterling, 'The Bare Bones of Sex: Part 1 – Sex and Gender', p. 1495.

12 Butler, *Bodies that Matter*, pp. xi–xii.

13 Ibid., p. 9, emphasis in original.

14 Linda Martín Alcoff, 'Philosophy Matters: A Review of Recent Work on Feminist Philosophy', *Signs*, 25:3 (2000), p. 858.

15 Karen Barad, 'Posthumanist Performativity: Toward an Understanding of How Matter Comes to Matter', *Signs*, 28:3 (2003), p. 810.

16 Donna Haraway, *When Species Meet* (Minneapolis, 2008), p. 4.

17 Barad, 'Posthumanist Performativity', pp. 823–824, emphasis in original.

18 Ibid., p. 802.

19 Ibid., p. 812.

20 Hans Schouwenburg, 'Back to the Future? History, Material Culture and New Materialism', *History, Culture and Modernity*, 3:1 (2015), pp. 63–64.

21 Anu Salmela, 'Fleshy Stories. New Materialism and Female Suicides in Late Nineteenth-Century Finland', *History, Culture and Modernity*, 6:1 (2018), p. 4.

22 Ibid., p. 10.

23 Ibid., p. 16.

24 Ibid., p. 17.

25 Karen Barad, 'Meeting the Universe Halfway: Realism and Social Constructivism without Contradiction', in Lynn Hankinson Nelson and Jack Nelson, eds, *Feminism, Science, and the Philosophy of Science* (Dordrecht/Boston, 1996), pp. 181, 219.

26 Keith Ansell-Pearson, 'Deleuze and New Materialism. Naturalism, Norms, and Ethics', in Sarah Ellenzweig and John H. Zammito, eds, *The New Politics of Materialism. History, Philosophy, Science* (London, 2017), pp. 88–108.

27 Ian Buchanan, 'The Problem of the Body in Deleuze and Guattari, or, What Can a Body Do?', *Body & Society*, 3:3 (1997), p. 76.

28 Gilles Deleuze and Félix Guattari, *A Thousand Plateaus*, translated by Brian Massumi (Minneapolis, 1987), p. 257.

29 Buchanan, 'The Problem of the Body in Deleuze and Guattari', p. 75.

30 Ibid., p. 80.
31 Ibid., p. 82.
32 Scott Lash, 'Genealogy and the Body: Foucault/Deleuze/Nietzsche', *Theory, Culture & Society*, 2:2 (1984), p. 15.
33 Deleuze and Guattari, *A Thousand Plateaus*, pp. 149–166; Buchanan, 'The Problem of the Body in Deleuze and Guattari', pp. 87–88.
34 Grosz, *Volatile Bodies*, pp. 168–170.
35 Buchanan, 'The Problem of the Body in Deleuze and Guattari', pp. 77–78.
36 Gilles Deleuze and Claire Parnet, *Dialogues*, translated by Hugh Tomlinson and Barbara Habberjam (London, 1987), pp. 110–111.
37 Branka Arsic, 'The Experimental Ordinary: Deleuze on Eating and Anorexic Elegance', *Deleuze and Guattari Studies*, 2 (supplement) (2008), pp. 34–59.
38 Lash, 'Genealogy and the Body: Foucault/Deleuze/Nietzsche', p. 9.
39 Grosz, *Volatile Bodies*, p. 180.
40 Laura Guillaume and Joe Hughes, eds, *Deleuze and the Body* (Edinburgh, 2011).
41 Lisa Helps, 'Body, Power, Desire: Mapping Canadian Body History', *Journal of Canadian Studies*, 41:1 (2007), pp. 129–130.
42 Ibid., p. 130.
43 Grosz, *Volatile Bodies*, p. 165.
44 Lash, 'Genealogy and the Body: Foucault/Deleuze/Nietzsche', p. 7.
45 Grosz, *Volatile Bodies*, p. 120.
46 Ibid.
47 Jon Roffe and Hannah Stark, 'Introduction: Deleuze and the Non/Human', in Idem, ed., *Deleuze and the Non/Human* (Basingstoke, 2015), p. 5.
48 Bruno Latour, *The Pasteurization of France*, translated by Alan Sheridan and John Law, (Cambridge, MA, 1988).
49 Bruno Latour, 'How to Talk About the Body? The Normative Dimension of Science Studies', *Body & Society*, 10 (2004), p. 206, emphasis in original.
50 Ibid., pp. 206–207, emphasis in original.
51 Ibid., p. 207.
52 Annemarie Mol, *The Body Multiple: Ontology in Medical Practice* (Durham, 2002), pp. 10–13.
53 Ibid., pp. 32–33.
54 Ibid., p. 43.
55 Ibid., p. 50, emphasis in original.
56 Ibid., p. 84.

57 Amade M'Charek, 'Beyond Fact or Fiction: On the Materiality of Race in Practice', *Current Anthropology*, 28:3 (2013), p. 430.

58 Ibid., p. 435.

59 Ibid., p. 424.

60 Alice Domurat Dreger, *Hermaphrodites and the Medical Invention of Sex* (Cambridge, MA, 1998), pp. 29–30.

61 Geertje Mak, *Inscriptions, Bodies and Selves in Nineteenth-Century Hermaphrodite Case Histories* (Manchester, 2012), pp. 229–232.

62 Geertje Mak, 'Doubting Sex from Within: A Praxiographic Approach to a Late Nineteenth-Century Case of Hermaphroditism', *Gender & History*, 18:2 (2006), p. 340.

63 Ibid., p. 341.

64 Ibid., p. 333.

65 Iris Clever and Willemijn Ruberg, 'Beyond Cultural History? The Material Turn, Praxiography, and Body History', *Humanities*, 35 (2014), p. 562.

66 Bruno Latour, 'Why Has Critique Run Out of Steam? From Matters of Fact to Matters of Concern', *Critical Inquiry*, 30:2 (2004), pp. 225–248; Sebastian Abrahamsson, Filippo Bertoni, Annemarie Mol and Rebeca Ibáñez Martín, 'Living with Omega-3: New Materialism and Enduring Concerns', *Environment and Planning D: Society and Space*, 33:1 (2015), pp. 4–19.

▶ Conclusion

1 Jonathan Reinarz and Kevin Siena, eds, *A Medical History of Skin: Scratching the Surface* (London, 2016); Emma L.E. Rees, *The Vagina: A Literary and Cultural History* (London, 2013).

2 Ava Baron and Eileen Boris, '"The Body" as a Useful Category for Working-Class History', *Labor*, 4:2 (2007), p. 24.

3 Roger Cooter, 'The Turn of the Body: History and the Politics of the Corporeal', *Arbor*, 186 (2010), p. 394.

4 Alain Corbin, Jean-Jacques Courtine and Georges Vigarello, 'Préface', in Idem, ed., *Histoire du corps*, part 1 'De la Renaissance aux Lumières' (Paris, 2005), p. 11.

5 Silvia Stoller, 'Phenomenology and the Poststructural Critique of Experience', *International Journal of Philosophical Studies*, 17:5 (2009), pp. 707–737.

6 Emma Dabiri, *Don't Touch My Hair* (London, 2019).

7 Sontag, *Illness as Metaphor*; Marjo Kaartinen, *Breast Cancer in the Eighteenth Century* (London, 2013); Barbara Ehrenreich, *Bright-sided. How Positive Thinking is Undermining America* (New York, 2009), pp. 15–44.

8 Ivan Crozier, 'Introduction. Bodies in History – The Task of the Historian', in Idem, ed., *A Cultural History of the Human Body in the Modern Age* (Oxford, 2010), pp. 23–24.

Glossary

Agency   The idea that individuals have the leeway to act, make decisions, and shape their own lives; with regard to the body: the ability to move and shape one's own body freely.

Agential realism   A term coined by physicist and new materialist Karen Barad, indicating a perspective on the world and knowledge practices that does not rely on binaries such as subject-object or nature-culture, but that assumes that all phenomena are 'material-discursive' and produced in 'intra-actions' between subject and object.

Alienation   In Marxist terminology, the estrangement of the individual workers from their labour products or from other people or nature, preventing them from realizing their full humanity. In feminist terminology the estrangement of women from male-dominated culture, women's sexual objectification, and their failure to realize their full potential.

Biopolitics/biopower   A term coined by Michel Foucault to indicate the techniques used by modern nation states to control and regulate their populations, especially in relation to health, illness, and productivity.

Cartesian dualism   The view of Descartes that body and mind are separate entities, in which the mind is privileged since it houses consciousness and rational thinking and leads the body.

Constructionism   The philosophical approach that argues that an entity (e.g., gender, race, or the body) varies in different periods and in different places and societies and hence is culturally constructed. This view is opposed to essentialist approaches, which emphasize that entities such as the body or sexual differences are biological and unchanging.

Cultural turn   A shift in the 1980s and 1990s in the focus of research in the humanities from politics and socio-economic structures to culture, informed by theories from anthropology, sociology, and cultural studies.

Degeneration   A concept from nineteenth-century social and biological sciences referring to the deterioration of the race, attested by the 'inferior' looks and bodies of the lower classes and non-white people.

Discourse   A term popularized by Michel Foucault, referring to the specific ways certain institutions or practices frame topics through language.

Discursive   see Discourse.

Dualism   see Cartesian dualism.

Embodiment   The lived body, or the body as it is experienced by individuals in relation to their cultural environment and other people.

Essentialism   The view that argues that an entity (e.g., gender, race, or the body) is natural and unchanging, as opposed to a social constructionist approach, which takes these entities to be culturally constructed and historically variable.

Existentialism   The philosophical approach that studies the human condition from the perspective of the acting, feeling, and living human individual. Best known from the French philosophers Jean-Paul Sartre and Simone de Beauvoir, existentialist thought highly values freedom and authenticity.

Gender   In feminist and gender studies, the term gender refers to the social and cultural construction of sexual differences. Gender is thus opposed to sex: gender means the social construction of masculinity and femininity in a certain place and time.

Habitus   A term popularized by Pierre Bourdieu, indicating an embodied, durable disposition that enables structured improvisation, or learned behaviour that becomes second nature.

Humoral theory   A body of ideas on the internal workings of the body, formulated by ancient authorities such as Hippocrates and Galen and remaining popular among doctors and laypeople in the West until the nineteenth century.

The theory assumed the existence of four fluids or humours (phlegm, black bile, yellow bile, and blood) dispersed unequally among people and influencing their character. An excess or deficit of these humours was thought to lead to disease.

Linguistic turn A shift in the focus of research in the humanities, based on the insight that meaning is made through language, representation, and discourse and informed by philosophy and literary studies.

Medicalization A term indicating the process by which human problems, whether mental or bodily, come to be seen and treated as medical conditions, and thus as objects of medical study, diagnosis, or treatment.

New materialism A theoretical paradigm that can be seen as a critique of the late twentieth-century dominance of the linguistic paradigm in the humanities, as well as a re-examination of the central place of the human being, focusing rather on the connections between humans and non-humans such as objects, animals, plants, and the environment. It thus foregrounds 'matter'. In addition, it seeks new theoretical approaches that go beyond discourse analysis.

Normalization A concept that in social theory refers to the construction of an idealized norm of conduct or body, which implies there is also an average and an aberration from the norm.

Perspectivalism The philosophical theory that states that all individuals have their own view on the world.

Phallocentrism The notion, popularized by feminist theory, that the phallus (the psychoanalytical concept referring to the penis and its symbolic connotations) is the central element in the organization of society; more generally it refers to the centrality of men in society.

Phenomenology The branch of philosophy that studies the structures of experience and consciousness, including the role of the body in human experience, taking a first-person view.

Phrenology A pseudo-science, developed in 1796 by the German physician Franz Joseph Gall, that claimed that a person's character could be discerned by examining the face and especially the skull.

Physiognomy   A pseudo-science, developed in the eighteenth century by the theologian, writer, and philosopher Johann Kasper Lavater, who claimed that character, intelligence, and emotions could be read from the shape of faces.

Postcolonialism   The academic study that critically analyzes the cultural legacy of colonialism in a decolonized world, especially colonialism's effects on global structures of inequality.

Posthumanism   Contemporary theories that emphasize that humans are no longer the centre of the world (a view called anthropocentrism), and instead viewing humans in relation to the environment, thus undermining traditional boundaries between the human, the animal, and technology.

Postmodernism   A worldview that, in the humanities and social sciences, is considered to include skepticism towards modern claims to objective knowledge and truth, as well as a focus on representation instead of reality. In historiography it is identified with the linguistic turn and its attention to language and discourse.

Poststructuralism   A body of thought presented by several French philosophers and literary theorists (most importantly Michel Foucault, Jacques Derrida, Julia Kristeva, and Roland Barthes) from the 1960s, centring on ideas such as the multiple interpretations of a text, representation, deconstruction of binary oppositions, and power. Poststructuralism is often seen as part of postmodernism.

Potentiality   A term derived from the philosophy of Gilles Deleuze, referring to the potential of the body: it views bodies as full of active desire to connect with other bodies.

Praxiography   An approach in the humanities and social sciences that focuses on practices in which knowledge is made, in contrast to discourses or representation. Praxiography's claim that different practices produce different bodies is a claim about ontology.

Psychoanalysis   A theory on the workings of the human mind developed from the 1890s onwards. Its founding father was Sigmund Freud. Psychoanalysis accords a central role to the unconscious, in particular unconscious human drives, such as sexual urges and aggression. Freud's model of the personality explained the human mind as consisting of ego, id, and super-ego: three contrasting elements, the id representing human drives, the super-ego the fatherly and cultural norms mostly forbidding these drives, and the ego that which is conscious in the person and represents the reality of the outside world to the self. Psychoanalysis has an eye for unconscious psychological conflicts, especially between personal, bodily desires and social taboos.

Psychosomatic A medical term referring to the interrelationship between mind and body in explaining disease, often implying that an illness in the body has psychological causes.

Representation A representation of the body is a portrayal of that body in text or image.

Social constructionism, see Constructionism.

Solidist Solidism is a late eighteenth-century theory on the workings of the body, focusing on the solid portions of blood vessels and nerves.

Somatic turn The new attention paid to the body paid in the humanities and social sciences from the 1980s and 1990s.

Somatization The expression of emotional or mental problems in bodily terms.

Structuralism A philosophical movement in the twentieth century that searched for structures in language to explain meaning, or structures in society to explain human behaviour, instead of designating individual agency as the primary mover. Famous structuralists include the linguist Ferdinand de Saussure and the anthropologist Claude Lévi-Strauss.

Technologies of the self A term coined by Michel Foucault to refer to those activities undertaken by individual subjects to shape their bodies, selves, emotions, and conduct to attain certain highly valued mental states.

Further Reading

▷ Introduction

The following articles provide clear overviews of the development of the field of body history: Kathleen Canning, 'The Body as Method? Reflections on the Place of the Body in Gender History', *Gender & History*, 11:3 (1999) pp. 499–513; Iris Clever and Willemijn Ruberg, 'Beyond Cultural History? The Material Turn, Praxiography, and Body History', *Humanities*, 35 (2014), pp. 546–566; Roger Cooter, 'The Turn of the Body: History and the Politics of the Corporeal', *ARBOR Ciencia, Pensamiento y Cultura*, 186: 743 (2010), pp. 393–405; Genevieve Galán Tamés, 'Aproximaciones a la Historia del Cuerpo Como Objeto de Estudio de la Disciplina Histórica', *Historia y Grafía*, 33 (2009), pp. 167–204. One of the first volumes published on body history as it was conceived by the linguistic and cultural turns is Catherine Gallagher and Thomas Laqueur, eds, *The Making of the Modern Body: Sexuality and Society in the Nineteenth Century* (Berkeley, 1987). More information on the cultural and linguistic turns can be found in Simon Gunn, *History and Cultural Theory* (Harlow, 2006) and Gabrielle Spiegel, 'Introduction' in idem ed., *Practicing History: New Directions in Historical Writing after the Linguistic Turn* (New York, 2005), pp. 1–34. A book that provides data on the physical changes of the body in modernity is Roderick Floud, Robert W. Fogel, Bernard Harris and Sok Chul Hong, *The Changing Body: Health, Nutrition and Human Development in the Western World since 1700* (Cambridge, 2011). The historical effects of industrialization on health are discussed by David Rosner and Gerald Markowitz, *Dying for Work: Workers' Safety and Health in Twentieth-Century America* (Bloomington, 1987). For further reading on the body in visual culture see: Sander L. Gilman, 'Black Bodies, White Bodies: Toward an Iconography of Female Sexuality in Late Nineteenth-Century Art, Medicine, and Literature', *Critical Inquiry*, 12:1 (1985), pp. 204–241.

▶ Chapter 1: Body, Mind, and Self: Historical Perspectives

An interdisciplinary, long-term history of how the human body has been understood in Europe is provided by John Robb and Oliver J.T. Harris, eds, *The Body in History: Europe from the Palaeolithic to the Future* (Cambridge, 2013). For an overview of the cultural history of the body, see Linda Kalof and William Bynum, eds, *A Cultural History of the Human Body*, 6 parts (Oxford, 2010); Fay Bound Alberti, *This Mortal Coil. The Human Body in History and Culture* (Oxford, 2016). For an overview of the history of sexuality, see Julie Peakman, *A Cultural History of Sexuality*, 6 parts (Oxford, 2010). Further reading on the body in antiquity includes: Anna Marmodoro and Sophie Cartwright, *A History of Mind and Body in Late Antiquity* (Cambridge, 2018); Helen King, *Hippocrates' Woman. Reading the Female Body in Ancient Greece* (London, 1998). For histories of the body in the Middle Ages, see Carolyn Walker Bynum, *Holy Feast and Holy Fast: The Religious Significance of Food to Medieval Women* (Berkeley, CA, 1987); Jack Hartnell, *Medieval Bodies* (London, 2018); Jacques Le Goff and Nicolas Truong, *Une Histoire du Corps au Moyen Âge* (Paris, [1983] 2012). A specific history of humoral theory is: Noga Arikha, *Passions and Tempers: a History of the Humours* (New York, 2008).

Helpful overviews of medical history include Jacalyn Duffin, *History of Medicine. A Scandalously Short Introduction*, 2nd edn (Toronto, 2010); Mary Lindemann, *Medicine and Society in Early Modern Europe*, 2nd edn (Cambridge, 2010); and Ian Miller, *Medical History* (London, 2018).

▶ Chapter 2: The Modern Body, Discipline, and Agency

A further comparison of Foucault and Elias can be found in Dennis Smith, 'The Civilizing Process and The History of Sexuality: Comparing Norbert Elias and Michel Foucault', *Theory and Society*, 28:1 (1999), pp. 79–100. Jana Sawicki, *Disciplining Foucault. Feminism, Power, and the Body* (New York, 1991) and Lois McNay, *Foucault and Feminism: Power, Gender and the Self* (Cambridge, 1992) discuss the ways Foucault's ideas on discipline and power can be applied to feminist approaches to the body. The edited volume by Colin Jones and Roy Porter, eds, *Reassessing Foucault: Power, Medicine and the Body* (London, 1994) contains chapters on how historians have applied Foucault's ideas on power and the body. An extensive discussion of the notion of 'biopolitics' can be found in Thomas Lemke,

Biopolitics: An Advanced Introduction (New York, 2011). On beauty practices and discipline, see Sander Gilman, *Making the Body Beautiful* (Princeton, NJ, 1999) and Idem, *Creating Beauty to Cure the Soul* (Durham, NC, 1998). The relationship between medicine, colonization, and the British empire is discussed in David Arnold, *Colonizing the Body: State Medicine and Epidemic Disease in Nineteenth-Century India* (Berkeley, 1993).

▶ Chapter 3: The Social Construction of the Body and Disease

Another introduction into social constructionist theories of the body can be found in Chris Shilling, *The Body & Social Theory*, 3rd edn (Los Angeles, CA, [1993] 2012), pp. 75–102. The use of the body as metaphor for social relations is discussed by Mary Poovey, *Making a Social Body: British Cultural Formation, 1830–1864* (Chicago, 1995); Frank Mort investigates how ideas on health and disease are connected to conceptions of sex and morality in *Dangerous Sexualities. Medico-Moral Politics in England since 1830*, 2nd edn (London, [1987] 2000). On the history of psychosomatic diseases, see Edward Shorter, *From Paralysis to Fatigue: A History of Psychosomatic Illness in the Modern Era* (New York, 1992). A recent overview of the history of mental illness is Petteri Pietikäinen, *Madness: A History* (London, 2015). The third chapter of Simon Gunn, *History and Cultural Theory* (Harlow, 2006) explores the influence of cultural anthropology on cultural history. A vast body of literature has been written on the history of hysteria, but a brief introduction is Andrew Scull, *Hysteria. The Disturbing History* (Oxford, [2009] 2011). Also see Sander L. Gilman, Helen King, Roy Porter, G.S. Rousseau, and Elaine Showalter, *Hysteria Beyond Freud* (Berkeley, CA, 1993). Further information on the history of anorexia can be found in Walter Vandereycken and Ron van Deth, *From Fasting Saints to Anorexic Girls. The History of Self-Starvation* (London, [1994] 1996). Michael Stolberg assesses social constructionism in regard to PMS in 'The Monthly Malady: A History of Premenstrual Suffering', *Medical History*, 44:3 (2000), pp. 301–322. The history of tuberculosis is explored in Helen Bynum, *Spitting Blood: The History of Tuberculosis* (Oxford, 2012). On the social construction of whiteness, see Noel Ignatiev, *How the Irish Became White* (London, 1995). On stereotypes, see Sander Gilman, *Difference and Pathology: Stereotypes of Sexuality, Race, and Madness* (Ithaca, 1985), and, on the cultural construction of the Jewish body, Sander Gilman, *The Jew's Body* (London, 1991).

A useful introduction to disability studies is Lennard J. Davis, *The Disability Studies Reader*, 5th rev. edn (London, 2017). More information on Sarah Baartman is found in Natasha Gordon-Chipembere, ed., *Representation and Black Womanhood. The Legacy of Sarah Baartman* (New York, 2011).

▶ Chapter 4: The Body, Gender, and Sexuality

On gender images in science, see Ludmilla Jordanova, *Sexual Visions. Images of Gender in Science and Medicine between the Eighteenth and Twentieth Centuries* (New York, 1989); Anne Fausto-Sterling, *Sexing the Body. Gender Politics and the Construction of Sexuality* (New York, 2000); Rebecca M. Jordan-Young, *Brainstorm. The Flaws in the Science of Sex Differences* (Cambridge, MA, 2010). Useful histories of sexuality and transgender persons include: Jeffrey Weeks, *Sex, Politics & Society. The Regulation of Sexuality Since 1800* (London, 1981); Dagmar Herzog, *Sexuality in Europe: A Twentieth-Century History* (Cambridge, 2011); Louis-Georges Tin, *The Invention of Heterosexual Culture* (Cambridge, MA, 2012); Isabel V. Hull, *Sexuality, State, and Civil Society in Germany*, 1700–1815 (Ithaca, NY, 1997); Thomas W. Laqueur, *Solitary Sex: A Cultural History of Masturbation* (New York, 2003); Judith Halberstam, *Female Masculinity* (Durham and London, 1998); Julian Gill-Peterson, *Histories of the Transgender Child* (Durham, NC, 2018); Rudolf M. Dekker and Lotte C. van de Pol, *The Tradition of Female Transvestism in Early Modern Europe* (London, 1989); Theo van der Meer, 'Tribades on Trial: Female Same-Sex Offenders in Late Eighteenth-Century Amsterdam', *Journal of the History of Sexuality*, 1:3 (1991), pp. 424–454; Martha Vicinus, *Intimate Friends: Women Who Loved Women, 1778–1928* (Chicago, 2004). Good introductions to gender theory and queer theory, respectively, are Laura Lee Downs, *Writing Gender History* (New York, 2004), and Nikki Sullivan, *A Critical Introduction to Queer Theory* (New York, 2003). For feminist sociological perspectives on the body, see Kathy Davis, ed., *Embodied Practices. Feminist Perspectives on the Body* (London, 1997).

▶ Chapter 5: Experiencing the Body

For more theoretical explorations of phenomenology and embodiment, see Thomas J. Csordas, ed., *Embodiment and Experience. The Existential Ground of Culture and Self* (Cambridge, 1994). The edited volume Paul Münch, ed., *"Erfahrung" als*

Kategorie der Frühneuzeitgeschichte (Munich, 2001) discusses the notion of experience as a category in early modern history. For a history of the senses, see Constance Classen, ed., *A Cultural History of the Senses* (London, 2014). A plea for the use of psychoanalysis in the cultural history of the body and emotion can be found in Michael Roper, 'Slipping Out of View: Subjectivity and Emotion in Gender History', *History Workshop Journal*, 59:1 (2005), pp. 57–72.

▶ Chapter 6: Materialist Approaches to the Body

A famous book addressing the influence of biology and disease in human history is Jared Diamond, *Guns, Germs, and Steel: The Fates of Human Societies* (New York, 1997). It is especially in the field of the history of emotions that the relationship between history and the neurosciences is discussed: see Ruth Leys, 'The Turn to Affect: A Critique', *Critical Inquiry*, 37:3 (2011), pp. 434–472, and William M. Reddy, *The Navigation of Feeling: A Framework for the History of Emotions* (Cambridge, 2001). For further reading on new materialism, see Diana Coole and Samantha Frost, eds, *New Materialisms: Ontology, Agency, Politics* (Durham, 2010); Rick Dolphijn and Iris van der Tuin, *New Materialism: Interviews & Cartographies* (Ann Arbour, MI, 2012).

Index

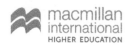
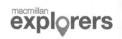

Access a library of eTextbooks for your history course, all in one place

Macmillan History Explorer

Using Macmillan Explorers you can...

Access offline on up to four devices

Save bookmarks

Print pages

Export notes & highligh to OneNote

Subscribe at **macmillanexplorers.com**